Withdrawn

TRANSITION
to
Vegetarianism

TRANSITION
to
Vegetarianism

An Evolutionary Step

RUDOLPH BALLENTINE, M.D.

The Himalayan Institute Press
Honesdale, Pennsylvania

© 1987, 1999 by The Himalayan International Institute
of Yoga Science and Philosophy of the USA
RR 1, Box 400
Honesdale, Pennsylvania 18431

8 7 6 5 4 3 2 1

Cover design by Jeanette Robertson

The paper used in this publications meets the minimum requirements of
American National Standard for Information Sciences–Permanence of
Paper for Printed Library Materials, ANSI Z39.48-1984.

Library of Congress Cataloging in Publication Data

Ballentine, Rudolph, 1941–
        Transition to vegetarianism.

        Includes index.
        I. Vegetarianism. II. Himalayan International Institute of Yoga Science and
Philosophy of the USA II. Title.
TX392.B297 1987   613.2'62   87–23618
ISBN 0–89389–175–4

CONTENTS

FOREWORD

The Himalayan International Institute is known for its synthesis of Eastern wisdom and Western science, which began in the 1960s with the work done by Swami Rama, the Institute's founder, at the Menninger Foundation. His demonstrations of the voluntary control of internal states established the groundwork for the development of biofeedback and an impetus for the extension of the holistic perspective into the field of health care.

Unfortunately the term "holistic" is often used to mask or to justify an attitude that is, in fact, anti-science and anti-rational. Many "alternative" practitioners have seriously impeded the development and wider acceptance of the holistic approach to health care by their uncritical and, at times, superstitious attachment to their work. In view of this, we owe Dr. Ballentine and his colleagues at the Himalayan Institute a great debt for their detailed and careful research. Their work and the publications arising out of it have been a healthy antidote to the unfortunate effects of much of what is passed off as holistic, and have provided the inspiration and guidance for clinical and teaching centers throughout the world.

This current volume on the benefits of a vegetarian diet is no exception. The understanding of the importance of diet to our physical well-being is finally becoming accepted. Dr. Ballentine, using an impressive array of evidence, suggests how our eating habits may affect our well-being. Time-honored Eastern traditional teachings on diet have been used to generate hypotheses which have been checked against computerized surveys of current research literature in the health sciences.

It is increasingly accepted that vegetarians do not suffer to the same degree from certain of the disease processes that affect meat-eaters so severely. Dr. Ballentine provides a critical analysis of meat-eating habits and demonstrates a thorough understanding of the potential harms and/or limitations on one's well-being from undesirable animal foods. The benefits to physical health of changing to a vegetarian diet are indisputably documented herein. Moreover, the probable benefit to mental life is strongly suggested.

But holistic health includes the physical, the mental, and the spiritual. The realization of one's potentials for spiritual growth depends on clarity of consciousness and a sharpened sense of self-awareness. Perhaps the most intriguing thesis that emerges from this book is that in addition to causing disease, the modern meat-based diet might dull one's awareness, limit one's capacity for creativity, and interfere with one's progress in the direction of personal evolution. Taken as a whole, the book firmly reinforces the age-old conviction that clarity and awareness are promoted by a vegetarian diet. If humankind is to evolve to its next step, the dimension of personal spiritual growth must be deepened and reinforced and a major means to this end may just turn out to be the transition to a vegetarian diet.

Dr. Patrick C. Pietroni, FRCGP, MRCP, DCH
Senior Lecturer in General Practice, St. Mary's
Hospital Medical School; Chair, British Holistic
Medical Association

PREFACE

In nearly twenty years of working with vegetarian patients and teaching them nutrition, I have come to be familiar with the questions most asked on the subject. When I set out to write this book, it was my purpose to provide a brief guide that would address these questions in a simple and straightforward way. But as I began a systematic survey of the scientific literature on vegetarianism, I came to realize that it had become much more extensive than I had thought.

Just in the last decade, a massive amount of evidence has accumulated which collectively provides an argument for the importance of moving toward a vegetarian diet—an argument so forceful as to compel the individual to modify his eating habits, and of proportions sufficient to mandate major changes in official attitudes and policies. With this in mind, I began to see the book as an opportunity to pull together and present as much as possible of this research so that its far-reaching implications might become more evident and more widely recognized. I hope that I have been able, at least to a modest extent, to accomplish this end.

As I reviewed and researched the literature, another basic point was repeatedly reinforced: dropping meat isn't enough. While the potential benefits of a vegetarian diet are profoundly impressive, the problems that can arise from doing it wrong are equally so. Zinc deficiency, for example, is a problem that may be considerably more widespread among vegetarians than is generally appreciated, and it deserves special attention, as do a number of other issues, such as that of iron or vitamin D. The book is intended to present the information most relevant to helping the reader move toward a vegetarian diet safely and wisely.

The format of the book also calls for a word of explanation. It's a common observation that most people make the transition to vegetarianism by way of a series of fairly predictable steps, dropping red meat first, poultry later, and eventually (sometimes) fish. The book is arranged to correspond to those steps in order to make it as convenient and usable as possible. At each step or phase the data that support the elimination of the food in question are first considered, and then the issues that arise as a result of dropping it are discussed, for example, how to get enough iron after red meat is stopped.

The parts of the book that bring to light certain little-known aspects of meat and poultry production, though entirely accurate, may be so shocking as to seem almost intentionally sensational. They have been included unabridged, however, because in many cases such facts must be thoroughly appreciated before one will feel justified in investing the considerable time and energy necessary to make fundamental changes in how he eats. Dietary habits are often deeply ingrained—especially those that have extended over generations and that may have become closely involved with family or ethnic identity.

It is hoped that the critique of meat and poultry detailed in the book will not preoccupy the reader nor distract him from the experience of optimism and excitement that can otherwise result from discovering the improved health, the increased sense of well-being, and the enhanced clarity of mind that follow the shift toward a well-balanced vegetarian diet. With more individuals enjoying such rewards, and with the weight of evidence so obviously supporting such dietary change, it seems inevitable that interest in it will spread. What awaits the reader is, I suspect, not only personal benefit but also the growing conviction that vegetarianism is likely to be the diet of the future—a logical next step in humankind's perennial search for a better way of living and being.

INTRODUCTION

When *Transition to Vegetarianism* was first published a dozen years ago, I predicted in the preface that more and more people would gravitate toward a vegetarian diet. That has certainly happened. Though some try vegetarianism for a while and then abandon it, a growing percentage of the population is taking a larger proportion of its food from non-animal sources.

The ecological crisis is making this shift ever more necessary and urgent. The fragile and weakening web of life that sustains us cannot bear the strain of producing enough meat to feed a burgeoning world population. Moreover, the level of environmental toxicity continues to increase at an alarming rate—at the time of this writing, for example, the United States produces close to a ton of petrochemicals per person per year. Because animals concentrate toxins in their bodies, eating primarily plant foods is becoming critically important in minimizing toxic intake. At the same time, the quality of conventionally raised livestock continues to deteriorate. Animals are in line for the same erosion of health as humans due to the pollution of the environment. Many researchers also think that the risk of repeating the British beef tragedy will continue to increase as long as we use the carcasses of sick animals to feed livestock destined for human consumption.

These are all potent reasons for moving toward a meatless diet. In addition, as is well-documented in the pages of this book, research suggests than even with healthy animals, a largely vegetarian diet minimizes the risk of heart disease, osteoporosis, arthritis, and other degenerative diseases. And there are other reasons, too. Even though this has not yet been studied in the laboratory, those sensitive to the subtler aspects of human functioning point out that the violence and suffering implicit in modern meat production may also have adverse effects on the mind and consciousness. Consuming such food has traditionally been seen as detrimental to emotional stability and mental clarity. Your consciousness, it is thought, absorbs and reflects the abuse of the animals you are eating.

There is no lack of evidence, on the other hand, that meat production is destructive to the ecology of the planet. The major reason the rain forest is being destroyed so rapidly is to create grazing land for beef cattle. This despite the fact that the amount of plant-based food that can be produced on an acre of land is many times what it will yield in meat.

In short, humanity can ill afford the use of animal foods when it must pay for that questionable luxury with increased toxicity, decreased health and well-being, and the waste of land, water, and food necessary to raise livestock. An animal-based diet is simply no longer feasible. To persist in demanding it would be irrational and self-destructive.

Fortunately, much of the world's population is grounded in traditions of low-meat diets. Developing countries do not need to repeat the tragic errors of their more affluent cousins. But they do need education in the risks of meat-eating and the benefits of a plant-based diet if those who are not yet habituated to animal-based diets are to strengthen their sounder dietary patterns and assume a position of leadership in creating a healthful diet for the future. This is not only possible, it has already begun, as indicated by the proliferation of ethnic restaurants and cookbooks—

from Thai to Middle Eastern—that lean heavily on low-meat or meat-free dishes from such cultures around the world.

When I visited China nearly a decade ago, I urged highly placed friends to slip a copy of *Transition to Vegetarianism* to the health ministry, in hopes that the impulse to imitate the West could be averted in the area of diet, and the goal of increasing meat consumption be recognized as the financial, ecological, and heath disaster that it would turn out to be. Unfortunately my efforts were unsuccessful, but awareness of these issues is increasing. When China applied to the World Bank for funding its planned livestock expansion, for example, the request was refused. The reason was not hard to guess. It was in China that pioneering and highly publicized nutritional research had been conducted showing that meat-eating was associated with increased incidences of cancer and other "diseases of civilization." Why fund an expensive project that would undermine health and create a demand for an ecologically unsound diet?

I remain optimistic that the information contained in this book can help chart a new course for agriculture and nutrition. Even in this age of information overload, when new research is exploding, the principles outlined herein have held up surprisingly well. *Transition to Vegetarianism* is as timely and trenchant today as when it was first published. Though additional evidence to support the concepts and conclusions presented here could be added, those concepts and conclusions stand essentially unchallenged.

This is because *Transition to Vegetarianism* is not based on a narrowly focused set of beliefs or habits, but on a cross-cultural comparison of the eating patterns of healthy cultures around the world. Dietary practices that popped up repeatedly in such a comparison were checked against current research, and when the scientific studies confirmed what the various traditions practiced, it became clear that there was a solid principle involved. For example, bean and grain dishes are a mainstay in the diet of almost every healthy population, and countless studies support the value of such a staple.

The three-phase process of moving first away from red meat, then poultry, and finally dropping either fish or dairy is an increasingly common feature of the nutritional landscape. The guidelines this book offers for taking those steps safely and sanely are needed more than ever. If there is anything that I wish I had included that I did not, it would be more emphasis on the value of feeling free to move back and forth between the different phases as one's needs and circumstances dictate. Though we will all, I believe, inexorably move in the direction of consuming less and less animal food, this process should not be forced or done mechanically.

We must respect our own limitations, the reality that we are embedded in a world that offers limited nutritional resources, and the fact that our actions affect the web of life which sustains us. It is, I believe, only by understanding the facts and having the benefit of a wider perspective that we will be able to help ourselves and others find the way to a healthier diet and a healthier planet.

Rudolph Ballentine, M.D.
May 1999

TRANSITION
to
Vegetarianism

WHY VEGETARIAN
. . . AND HOW

As recently as the early 1960s, diets without meat were considered the domain of the eccentric, the bizarre, or the deranged. But now, ideas are changing rapidly. In recent years "vegetarian" has become a household word. Flight attendants on airlines routinely handle requests for vegetarian meals, and restaurants having any interest at all in appearing up-to-date must have vegetarian alternatives listed on their menus. Food sections in major newspapers carry frequent articles on meatless recipes, while cookbooks catering to vegetarians are selling briskly. According to a poll, in 1985 over six million Americans called themselves vegetarians. A popular news magazine terms vegetarianism "very much middle-class mainstream."

Why all the commotion about an idea that is anything but new? A recent survey by the United States Department of Agriculture found that two thirds of households had made changes in their diets "for reasons of health or nutrition," and that households with higher educational levels were more likely to change their diets. The changes reported included a decrease in beef and pork and an increase in vegetables. In fact, Americans are eating 11% more vegetables and 7% more fruits than five years ago.

There's a new trend afoot today in attitudes toward diet. It

3

involves making choices consciously rather than following ethnic or cultural traditions blindly. Up to now, the dietary habits of most people in the world have been largely shaped by imitating family patterns of eating. Attitudes toward food were deeply ingrained and often resistant to change.

By contrast, today's revolution in ideas about diet involves a growing awareness of the relationship between how one eats, on the one hand, and one's health and well-being, on the other. There is an increasing effort to make informed decisions and to base dietary practices on reason and good sense, rather than on emotion or past conditioning. This provides an unprecedented opportunity for improving health. A sense of that potential seems to fill the air, bringing optimism, enthusiasm, and the creative energy needed to examine old habits and to make constructive changes.

Vegetarianism no longer smacks of penance or self-denial. It is definitely upbeat. Meatless meals are seen as part of an active, exuberant lifestyle—one that is both youthful and responsible.

Vegetarianism and Social Awareness

Vegetarianism is also advocated by those concerned with the economic pressure of feeding the world's burgeoning population. From the perspective of land use and the efficiency of agriculture, producing meat is much more expensive than producing vegetable foods. A beef cow must be fed 21 pounds of plant protein in order to produce 1 pound of animal protein for human consumption. Fully one half of all the agricultural land in use in the United States is planted with feed crops, most of which are used to produce meat.[1] Our livestock consumes 10 times the amount of grain we eat ourselves.[2]

This means that a great deal of protein is wasted by feeding it to animals and then eating them, rather than using the plant food directly. Though this same pattern is common in many of the developed countries of the world, the United States is the most extreme example. It has been estimated that with what we waste in our country alone, through meat consumption, 90% of the protein deficit for the entire world could be met. If meat were dropped from the diets of the U.S. and a few other countries, everyone on earth could eat well.

These figures are based on grain consumption, and grain is not even the most efficient use of land for protein production. Though an acre of cereals can produce 5 times as much protein as an acre devoted to livestock, legumes (beans and peas) can produce 10 times as much. Leafy vegetables will yield even more. Spinach, for example, will provide more than 25 times as much protein from an acre of land as will beef.

Such facts have made it clear that feeding the hungry people of the earth not only is feasible but could be greatly facilitated by a change of dietary habits among the meat-eaters of the developed countries. As the population of the world soars, the ration of arable land per person drops. In some areas the situation is critical. A commission of the National Academy of Sciences concluded that in order to survive, we must learn to rely more on plants and less on meat for our nourishment.[3]

There are other reasons, too, for the vegetarian alternative. Many people find it unappealing or morally objectionable to eat flesh foods because to do so necessitates killing animals. Although decisions about diet based on concerns for health or the global economy are part of a new consciousness, there have long been those opposed to taking the lives of animals to secure food, and the list of "ethical vegetarians" is lengthy. Some of history's most outstanding figures have been vegetarians, many for reasons of avoiding the slaughter of animals. They include Leo Tolstoy, H. G. Wells, Albert Einstein, George Bernard Shaw, Albert Schweitzer, Mahatma Gandhi, Henry David Thoreau, Ralph Waldo Emerson, Richard Wagner, Charles Darwin, Benjamin Franklin, Voltaire, Sir Isaac Newton, Leonardo da Vinci, William Shakespeare, and, in early Rome and Greece, Virgil, Horace, Plato, and Pythagoras.

Of course vegetarianism has also been the rule rather than the exception among the world's great spiritual teachers. Buddha is the preeminent example; some scholars of early Christianity claim that Jesus also was explicitly vegetarian.[4] Verses in both the

Old and New Testaments of the Bible as well as passages in the Koran and various sacred scriptures of the Hindus[5] warn against consuming flesh foods. Nevertheless, over the centuries, vegetarianism for moral reasons has been regarded, by and large, as extreme and ill-advised.

Among the population masses of the countries of the West a meatless diet has historically been considered to be risky business from the point of view of health. If one stopped at all to wonder how the George Bernard Shaws of the world managed to survive on a vegetarian diet, one probably concluded that they ate a bit of meat on the sly—enough to stay alive, anyhow. It was widely believed that a diet without meat was inadequate to supply one's basic needs. But it is probably this idea about vegetarianism that has changed most dramatically. In fact, the most popular and appealing argument for a vegetarian diet today has to do with its health benefits. For that reason we shall explore in depth the impact a vegetarian diet has on health and disease.

THE VEGETARIAN DIET AND HEALTH

It has been only a decade or two since the scientific community began to consider the possibility that a vegetarian diet could be as healthful as one that contains meat. The earliest hint of such a change in attitude came in the early 1950s when a group of nutritionists at Harvard published the first systematic study in this country on vegetarianism. Since at the time Seventh-Day Adventists constituted one of the few populations that followed a vegetarian diet with any consistency, a group of them was used as subjects. All had been vegetarian for a minimum of five years. About half were adolescents and pregnant women; they were included because their nutritional requirements are high and an inadequate diet could be expected to produce signs of deficiency in them most quickly. Dietary histories were used to compute nutrient intakes, and all subjects underwent a thorough physical examination including a careful measurement of height, weight, and blood pressure. Laboratory tests for anemia, cholesterol, and blood proteins were done.[6-8] The pregnant women were followed through delivery so that data on their infants could be collected.

On all counts the vegetarians were normal. In fact, their blood cholesterol levels were better than those of meat-eaters, and an analysis of their dietary histories showed their intake of vitamins and other essential nutrients to be quite adequate.

These results were different from what had been expected. Those who felt confident about the value of meat in the diet suggested that perhaps the Seventh-Day Adventists were healthy because they didn't smoke or drink. Certainly there was no rush to embrace vegetarianism. It had long been a part of nutritional orthodoxy that good-quality protein could come only from meat. Vegetable proteins were "incomplete"—not adequate for sustaining life. Experiments using diets based on individual vegetable foods tended to support this thinking.

A giant step forward came, however, with the publication in 1971 of a little book called *Diet for a Small Planet,* which brought to the public's attention a simple nutritional fact that had been largely overlooked. Written by someone who was neither nutritionist nor laboratory scientist, it pointed out that vegetable foods taken in the proper combinations could supply protein of a quality equal to that of meat. This was not a maneuver that required strange dietary practices. As it turned out, such combinations of vegetable foods had been, and still are, staples for many people around the world who eat little meat, and provide the basic protein in their diets.

Nevertheless, with this key concept more widely acknowledged, moving toward a vegetarian diet seemed safer, and as vegetarians began to appear on the scene in greater numbers and were available to study, scientific articles validating the adequacy of a vegetarian diet emerged.[9-11] In fact, as the data accumulated, it became increasingly evident that not only is a vegetarian diet adequate, but in many respects it is more conducive to good health than the usual diet consumed by Americans. Does this mean vegetarians are healthier? Actually, the more statistics pile up, the more it looks as though that may be the case. As vegetarians are studied with increasing frequency and thoroughness, they are found to be less prone to a number of those diseases that are most serious and prevalent today.

Much of the rest of this book will be devoted to looking at specific aspects of the vegetarian diet, and how each of these provides protection against various disorders. For example, we will examine the mineral content of vegetable foods and how it affects the incidence of osteoporosis. We will also discuss in some detail which types of fiber can decrease blood cholesterol levels. But at this point it might provide a helpful orientation for the reader if we step back for a moment and survey the field as a whole, to get a general overview of the effects on health and disease that have been correlated with a meat-free diet. In the next chapter we will cover some of the same territory again, in an attempt to define more precisely what it is in the vegetarian diet that is responsible for each of these benefits.

Heart Disease

An impressive example of the benefits of a vegetarian diet is its effect on coronary heart disease. Any measure that can help to prevent this disease deserves attention, since heart disease may well be the greatest health problem in America today. It is responsible for more than 550,000 deaths each year in this country.[12] In addition, there are more than 5.4 million Americans whose

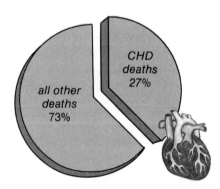

Percentage of All Deaths in the U.S. Due to Coronary Heart Disease (CHD) in 1985

Source: National Heart-Lung Institute.[12]

lives are limited by the symptoms of heart disease, and there are large numbers of others with the disease who are as yet un-diagnosed. It has been estimated that coronary heart disease costs the U.S. more than $60 billion annually.

Vegetarians have lower levels of certain risk factors for heart disease, such as total serum cholesterol, [13-21] triglycerides, [19-21] and low-density lipoproteins. [16,17,20-22,nt.1] An improvement in risk factors should mean less heart disease. As early as 1961 one physician was bold enough to write in the *Journal of the American Medical Association* that "97% of coronary occlusions [the usual heart attacks] could be prevented by a vegetarian diet." At that time there was little evidence to back up such a statement, but over the years a number of research papers have been published that put this claim on an increasingly solid foundation in fact. Some of them have looked directly at heart disease in vegetarians and found it to be decreased, [15,20,23-25] while others provide supporting data.[26-29]

One recently completed study of 25,000 Californians carried out over a 20-year period showed that meat consumption was associated with a higher incidence of fatal heart attacks in both men and women. Elaborate statistical analyses indicated that these effects were not due to differences in exercise habits between the vegetarians and those who were not vegetarian, nor were they due to differences in tobacco use, obesity, or the consumption of other foods besides meat and poultry. The results suggest a dose-response relationship between meat consumption and heart disease: the more meat eaten, the more heart disease. The difference was most pronounced in men of middle age. For men 45 to 64, there were more than three times as many fatal heart attacks in those who ate meat and poultry than there were in those who were vegetarian.[25]

The beneficial effects on the health of the heart alone should be enough to motivate many people to embark on the transition to vegetarianism, since heart disease, despite some recent decrease in frequency, is still the number one cause of death in America. Of course, one should not conclude that heart disease is due solely to diet, or that dietary change alone can prevent it totally. Many

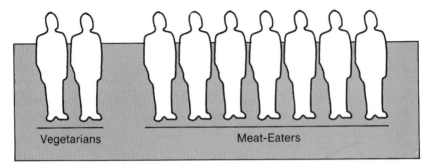

Rate of Fatal Heart Attacks in Vegetarians and Meat-Eaters
(Men, Ages 45 to 64)

Source: Snowdon, Phillips, & Fraser: *Meat Consumption.*[25]

other factors have been conclusively shown to contribute to its development, foremost among them cigarette smoking, lack of proper exercise, and high blood pressure.

But it now seems likely that diet can also play a role in the prevention or improvement of high blood pressure. This conclusion emerges from a variety of studies that have looked at the relationship between vegetarianism and blood pressure from a number of different angles. For example, vegetarians have repeatedly been found to have lower blood pressures than those who eat meat,[14] though this difference is probably less dramatic for those who use milk and eggs,[30-32] and adding meat to the diets of vegetarians raises their blood pressure.[13] Vegetarians also develop abnormally high blood pressure (hypertension) much less often than meat-eaters: only 2% of vegetarians, compared with 26% of nonvegetarians in one study.[33] Moreover, putting meat-eaters who are hypertensive on a vegetarian diet—even when the diet contains milk and eggs, and salt intake is not reduced—still results in a small but significant decrease in blood pressure.[34] And finally, diets that are essentially vegetarian have been the basis of a number of treatment programs designed to treat hypertension or reverse coronary heart disease.[35-37]

Both in terms of its direct effects on heart disease and the indirect benefits that follow reduction in blood pressure, the vegetarian diet seems to hold great promise as a major weapon in the battle against death and disability from cardiovascular disease.

Cancer

Not far behind heart disease, and gaining ground, is cancer. Cancer, like heart disease (or, for that matter, almost any other disease), probably results from a variety of causal factors acting in concert, but it has been estimated that the portion of total cancer in the United States that is significantly related to diet is 60% for women and 40% for men.[38] There is a growing consensus that cancer rates are lower in vegetarians, especially cancer of the breast and colon,[39,40] which are among the most common forms of cancer in the United States. In fact, until quite recently, colon cancer, which is almost unknown in those who eat a healthful vegetarian diet, was the most common malignancy in this country. Though recently surpassed in frequency by lung cancer, which is closely tied to smoking, colon cancer remains a major cause of death.

Several excellent research studies have found cancer of the colon to be positively correlated with foods of animal origin.[41-46] For example, in Argentina and Uruguay, where meat consumption is higher than it is in the rest of South America, colon cancer is more prevalent.[40] Evidence suggests that a vegetarian diet probably helps to prevent this disease[39] as well as cancer of the breast.[35]

Cancer of the prostate is less frequent in those whose diets are lower in fats and protein and richer in vegetables,[47] both of which are true of vegetarians. It is encouraging to think that the incidence of these three diseases, which together make up a large portion of the cancer occurring in the United States today, could be significantly reduced by the transition to a vegetarian diet.

Other Diseases

Diabetes, another major health problem, is also less frequent in those who consume diets that emphasize rice, beans, and vegetables, the basic components of a vegetarian diet.[48] Moreover, a largely vegetarian diet has produced surprising improvements in many diabetics,[36,49] especially in those with the milder adult-onset form of the disease. Such a diet has also been helpful for those who have other problems with blood sugar regulation, such as hypoglycemia.[50-52]

Vegetarians also have a lower incidence of a number of other common and troublesome diseases, such as osteoporosis[53,54] (see Phase 2), diverticulosis and diverticulitis,[55,56] gallstones[56,57] and even constipation.[8] What's more, most of the data available indicate that vegetarians tend to be slimmer and closer to desirable weights than nonvegetarians.[11,21,58,59] This is important, since obesity is an established risk factor for both heart disease and some forms of cancer[60,61] as well as being a common cause for concern in and of itself.

To sum up, it is beginning to appear that a vegetarian diet holds the potential for preventing disease on a scale that is far beyond what one might have imagined. Why would this be so? As research in the area becomes more sophisticated, it is clear that there are many facets to this question. As we shall see in subsequent sections of this book, a well-balanced, largely vegetarian diet, rich in whole grains, beans, vegetables, and fruits, corrects a number of serious defects in the current American diet.

What Is a Good Diet?

A good diet must include adequate protein for building tissues and other body components and an adequate intake of fuel to supply the energy needed to run the metabolic machinery. Either carbohydrate or fat can be burned, but all evidence suggests that carbohydrate is preferable for the bulk of energy needs and that simple carbohydrate (sugar) should comprise only a small portion of this. Probably very little fat is needed as long as what is present is of good quality.

The ratio of protein to carbohydrate should be close to 1 to 10. The amount of fuel needed will depend on how active one is, but the average person will do quite well on 1,800 to 2,500 calories.

A wide array of micronutrients, those needed in only very

small amounts, are also required in the diet. These are vitamins and minerals, and are the nuts and bolts used in setting up the metabolic machinery that can't be manufactured inside the body.

Of course, unless we are consuming an experimental diet, we are unlikely to pile our plates with servings of carbohydrate, fat, protein, or vitamins. We eat plant and animal products, and for the most part these contain an assortment of proteins, carbohydrates, and micronutrients. Most plant foods also contain fiber, which though not generally digested or absorbed is nevertheless important in the diet.

Nutritional requirements can therefore be described in two basic ways: in terms of individual nutrients—protein, carbohydrate, or vitamins, for example—or in terms of intact common foods—such as meat, grains, green and yellow vegetables, or dairy products. Talking about dietary requirements in terms of foods is more practical and commonsensical, but analysis of nutrients can reveal excesses or deficiencies that may have been overlooked and that may have serious consequences.

The typical American diet is extraordinarily high in fats and oils, due to the heavy use of meat, poultry, fish, cheese, frying oils, salad dressing, mayonnaise, pastries, and snack foods. Sugar and salt intake is quite high. The average American in 1900 took twice as much complex carbohydrate (starch) from foods such as grains and vegetables as he did sugar; now that ratio has been reversed: sugars exceed starches two to one. It is well recognized now that such large amounts of sugar can disturb glucose metabolism, elevate blood fats, and place added stress on metabolic systems. Borderline or inadequate intakes of several vitamins and minerals are common.[nt.2] As shall be explained in some detail in the remainder of this book, the vegetarian diet helps to correct a number of these problems.[63] It provides less fat, more complex carbohydrate, and a more optimal quota of vitamins and minerals. A vegetarian diet also furnishes a generous supply of fiber—one of its major advantages over a typical American meat-based diet. Current intakes of fiber are quite low, while the intake of food additives and chemicals from the environment is high. As we are about to see, this is not a happy combination.

Environmental Toxins and the Vegetarian Diet

Plants are the basis of all human nutrition. Meat is second-hand, in a sense: it is formed as a result of animals consuming plants. Next in this chain are those who eat meat, such as carnivorous mammals or birds of prey. Environmental toxins are progressively concentrated as one moves up the food chain.

This happens because animals eating contaminated plants gradually accumulate the toxic materials contained in the plants. By using animals for food, the carnivores who are next up in this sequence find themselves on a diet that contains higher levels of the toxic substances, and as these carnivores accumulate what is present in their prey, concentrations in their tissues gradually rise well above those of the animals they eat.

For example, hawks and eagles that live on the flesh of small animals have suffered a reduction in numbers because their eggs would not hatch. This is thought to be due to pesticide residues in the egg.[65] An animal eating a carnivore, being another step further up on the food chain, would be in danger of developing even higher levels of poison in its body. It's perhaps for this reason that humans have usually avoided using flesh-eating birds or animals as a source of food. This provides some protection against the intake of toxic substances—man-made or naturally occurring—that can accumulate in food chains.

A meat-free diet is even more protective, because eating a predominantly vegetarian diet allows one to eat still lower on the food chain. This is of particular significance if one is concerned about toxic chemicals such as pesticides that may be taken in through the diet.

Pesticides have been used extensively in homes and factories, but because current agricultural practices rely heavily on the use of insecticides and herbicides, their presence in food supplies has been a matter of special concern. Rachel Carson first called attention to the problem in 1962 in her book *Silent Spring*. Yet the use of agricultural pesticides in the United States has increased from 200,000 pounds per year in the 1950s to 1.1 billion pounds today. Fortunately, according to a recent news report, less than 2% of plant foods tested are above the suggested tolerance levels for residues.[66] Animal foods, on the other hand, reflect their position on the food chain and their tendency to concentrate chemicals from the plants or animals they eat: pesticide levels in them are considerably higher (see figure below).

DDT and DDT Derivatives as an Example of Pesticide Residues in Common Canadian Foods

Values given in micrograms per 100 grams.

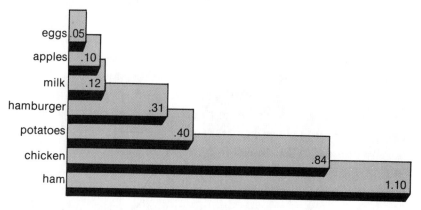

eggs	.05
apples	.10
milk	.12
hamburger	.31
potatoes	.40
chicken	.84
ham	1.10

Source: Coffin & McKinley: *Sources of Pesticide Residues.*[67]

Insecticides are of two major classes: chlorinated hydrocarbons, typified by DDT, and organophosphates, which have been used as nerve poisons in chemical warfare and which have been marketed recently under such names as malathion.

DDT, like the other chemicals in its class, is a relatively stable compound, so it persists for quite a long time. After crops are sprayed with it, it will turn up in the soil or food supplies years later. DDT and the other chlorinated hydrocarbon pesticides had been discontinued or severely restricted by the end of the 1970s. Though they have now been replaced by less persistent chemicals that do not tend to accumulate in the environment, residues of them still turn up. Since they are fat soluble, they are especially high in foods containing animal fats. Yet studies do show that their levels are decreasing, and over a period of years they should slowly disappear from our food supplies.[67] The newer organophosphates such as malathion, shorter-lived but perhaps more toxic, have been found in vegetable oils and in oranges and apples, but levels have been well within the limits of what is considered safe.[67]

More troublesome in a way than the pesticides are the notorious PCBs and PBBs—industrial chemicals that have escaped into the environment. They are not biodegradable at all and are therefore even more persistent than DDT, tending to float about in the air, water, and food supply indefinitely. Moreover, they are toxic at considerably lower doses than DDT.

The United States Food and Drug Administration set a maximum permissible PCB level of five parts per million in fish. But breastmilk of mothers living in industrial areas has commonly shown levels this high and higher.[68] Like DDT and other similar compounds, PCBs accumulate in food chains, so there is concern about their cumulative toxicity. Exposure to high doses has led to an increased rate of liver cancer,[69] but experts feel that at the levels usually present PCBs do not in and of themselves make a major contribution to the incidence of cancer in the population at large. There remains, nevertheless, the possibility that they might act synergistically with other cancer-causing agents and thereby increase risk.[70]

PBBs (polybrominated biphenyls) are similar compounds that came dramatically into the news as a result of the "Firemaster incident" in Michigan in 1973. A truck driver accidentally delivered to a manufacturer of animal feeds 2,000 pounds of a fire retardant based on PBBs, instead of the expected magnesium supplement. The fire retardant containing the toxic chemical was added to the feed and distributed to hundreds of farms in Michigan. As a result, thousands of animals died and there have been disturbing levels of PBBs in the Michigan food supplies for some years. Fortunately the Firemaster disaster was a local one, and, unlike PCBs, PBBs are not widespread environmental contaminants.

Other environmental toxins of concern that find their way into the food supply are those that are present primarily in meat, such as DES, which will be discussed in the next chapter, and the heavy metals, such as lead and mercury. Mercury is a problem restricted primarily to fish and will be dealt with later, but lead is much more pervasive, and lead poisoning is thought to be quite common. This is especially true in inner cities, where automobile exhaust fumes from leaded gasoline are concentrated. In American cities, one of every four children is thought to be suffering from lead toxicity.[71] Affecting preferentially the nervous system, lead causes emotional and behavioral problems, and eventually brain damage.

Because of the widespread distribution of lead in the environment that has occurred in modern times, lead is found at varying levels in the food supply. It accumulates in bone and as a rule is highest in animal foods that may contain some bone fragments, such as hamburger. However, shellfish taken from polluted waters have on occasion been found to have extremely high levels.[72] Plant foods generally have little, though wild greens gathered along busy highways may have dangerous levels of lead picked up from automobile exhaust.

Fiber and the Removal of Toxic Substances

With so many notes of alarm sounded by the news media about environmental toxins, it is easy to lose one's perspective on the matter. Actually, as we have seen, there are a number of frequently mentioned substances that at the present time pose no widespread or serious threat. Those that are still of considerable concern are primarily PCBs, lead, and mercury. A vegetarian diet may offer significant protection from all of them.

A diet made up predominantly of plant foods not only decreases one's intake of many toxic substances, because it entails eating low on the food chain, but may be protective in another way, too: research suggests that fiber, the undigested component of plant foods, may absorb and carry out of the body a variety of chemicals, drugs, and food additives that would otherwise be absorbed. Young rats fed a toxic dose of red dye and a low-fiber diet stopped growing and died within two weeks. Various combinations of nutritional supplements didn't help. But when leafy plant foods were added to the diet, the toxic effects were counteracted.[73]

It would appear that some toxic substances in food can be held to a large extent by the plant fiber and carried out with the stool.

Which toxic substance is absorbed probably depends on the particular fiber constituents present in the plant (see pp. 194-201). This protective effect appears to be absent when the same chemicals are present in a highly refined diet, such as one made up predominantly of animal foods, white flour, sugar, fats, and oils. A vegetarian diet, rich in vegetables, fruits, grains, and beans and containing a variety of fiber types, should provide maximal protection. It has been shown, for example, that the pesticide level in the milk of nursing mothers was lower in those who were vegetarian.[74]

Moreover, a diet rich in high-fiber fruits, vegetables, grains, and beans also has a beneficial effect on the condition and

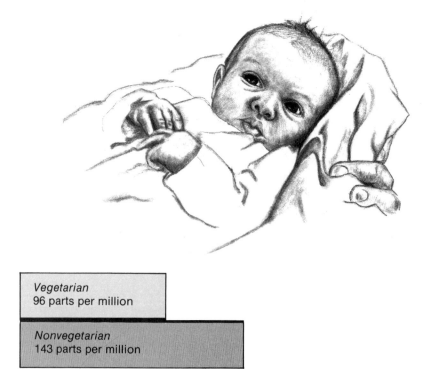

Vegetarian
96 parts per million

Nonvegetarian
143 parts per million

Averaged Levels of Pesticides and PCBs in Milk from Nursing Mothers with Different Diets

Source: Noren: *Levels of Organochlorine Contaminants.*[74, nt.3]

functioning of the gastrointestinal tract, as well as having the numerous other positive effects that will be described in more detail in later chapters of this book. For all these reasons, as long as the diet is properly designed so that deficiencies don't develop, the effects of a largely vegetarian diet should add up to significant improvements in health.

BEYOND HEALTH: STRENGTH, ENDURANCE, AND CLARITY OF CONSCIOUSNESS

There is a growing awareness that building health not only prevents untold suffering and expense but also has its more positive side: being healthy feels better and permits one to do more, to be more active, and to enjoy life more fully. In order to contribute to the development of health of this sort, an optimal diet should not only prevent disease, it should increase one's strength and stamina.

Although today one might think of vegetarians as lean, light, and airy—even energetic, after a fashion—they're apt to be considered a bit wanting in the area of strength and endurance. One who wishes to be strong eats meat—or at least that's our collective image. The training tables of football teams groan under the weight of beef roasts and pork chops. To feed them otherwise would be courting defeat, right?

Wrong. Perhaps one of the best-kept secrets in the area of athletics is the surprising effects of a vegetarian diet on performance. Just after the turn of the century, experiments done in Europe and later confirmed in America produced results in exact contradiction to popular notions about athletic prowess and diet.[75] The American studies, done at Yale in 1907, pitted meat-eaters against vegetarians in a deep knee bending contest. Only one of the meat-eaters could reach the 1,000 mark, whereas six of those on the largely vegetarian diet were able to do so. In fact, two of the six vegetarians managed 2,000 repetitions each.[76] A few similar tests have been done in recent decades looking at the more immediate effects of diet on endurance. In 1968 a Danish researcher found that for men on an average mixed diet, shifting to meat, milk, and eggs for three days cut endurance in half, whereas a purely vegetarian diet *increased* it by 50%.[77]

Although disappointingly little research has been done to follow up on these landmark studies, records set by vegetarian athletes are far out of proportion to their numbers. In 1956, a 17-year-old swimmer named Murray Rose became the world's youngest Olympic triple gold medal winner. He came back in 1960 to win further gold and silver medals, retaining his 400 meter title and becoming the first Olympic swimmer ever to do so. Later, he broke his own records and is considered one of the greatest swimmers of all time. He was a vegetarian.[78] Other famous swimmers such as Johnny Weismuller, of Tarzan fame, have set multiple world records after following a vegetarian diet.

Not only swimmers, but vegetarian football players, basketball players, and even weight lifters have had distinguished careers.[79,80] In the East these facts are not considered surprising. Observations of nature provide clues to the effects of diet. In the classic fight between the elephant and the lion, the elephant always prevails. Though more aggressive and ferocious, the carnivorous lion lacks both the strength and the endurance of the vegetarian elephant. Long after the lion collapses in exhaustion the elephant stands alert and ready to continue.

A well-designed vegetarian diet not only increases strength and endurance, it also has been felt to clear the head. Many persons have spontaneously observed that a progressive decrease of meat in their diet has led to a greater clarity of consciousness. They value the relative alertness, calmness, and sense of equanimity that seem to accompany a meat-free diet. So far, little research has been done to explore such subjective observations. Nevertheless, it is intriguing to note that for millennia the elimination of meat has been an important facet of many great spiritual traditions. It is almost a universal teaching that eliminating meat from the diet leads to a greater capacity for prayer, meditation, and self-awareness.

There is, moreover, a close correlation between cultivating health and expanding and sharpening awareness. The two pursuits go hand in hand because they work together so synergistically. A healthier person is better able to be calm and alert because he's less distracted by illnesses and discomforts. A person who cultivates alertness and awareness is better able to understand his body, regulate it, and increase his level of health.

THE TRANSITION PLAN

Regardless of whether the reader still eats meat on a regular basis or has already taken steps toward eliminating it, an important question arises at this point: How can we go about making such a change wisely? That is one of the major issues this book will address.

The successful cultivation of better health and increased awareness always occurs in a gradual manner, which is an important point to remember in making dietary modifications. This book is entitled *Transition to Vegetarianism,* and advisedly so. Shifting from a primarily meat diet to one that is mostly vegetarian is a drastic move. It should be made in a slow, gradual fashion.

A sudden change in the diet can be experienced as a disabling shock. Such jolts might produce dramatic effects, but on the whole they are undesirable: violent action produces a violent reaction. The body needs time to regear itself to deal with a different food supply. When the shift in diet is too abrupt, constructive adaptation is not possible.

This concept has become current in the area of stress research. Any organism can deal with change comfortably as long as it is of a certain magnitude. Past that limit, however, the inducement to change is no longer responded to positively, with a comfortable and appropriate adaptation. Instead, it becomes a cause for alarm. The autonomic nervous system, for example, is aroused to prepare for emergency action. The physiological events that ensue are those normally designed to deal with a threat to the organism's integrity and survival. When such a stress reaction follows an abrupt shift in diet, the benefits that might otherwise accrue from a potentially helpful change will be obscured by sudden and drastic disruptions of function.

You Are How *You Eat, Too*

Not only are such reactions physical, they can be psychological as well. There is a close correspondence between habits of diet and habits of mind and body. Eating in a certain fashion sustains the mental, emotional, and physiological patterns that are characteristic of us. How much one eats, for example, affects one's mood and alertness. Even modest overeating (which is far from uncommon) creates a certain dulling or sedative effect. When this becomes habitual, one comes to organize one's activities, relationships, and expectations around it. A mild degree of after-dinner stupor, prevented from degenerating into frank sleep by a timely cup of coffee, may come to be counted on as an antidote to the pressures of a busy day. To discontinue such habits abruptly is to create a sense of uncertainty and often anxiety.

Entire complexes of such habits—overeating, the excessive use of fats and oils from rich and fried foods and from large portions of high-fat meats, and the consumption of large quantities of sugar, along with the custom of taking alcoholic beverages, tobacco, and caffeine to magnify or counteract the effects of the diet—all have a powerful impact on the functioning of both body and mind. The regular, recurrent, and eventually characteristic modes of functioning that develop in conjunction with these dietary patterns are what psychologists call personality.

One psychiatrist, who became deeply involved with holistic therapies and increasingly convinced of the importance of diet, found himself frustrated by his unsuccessful attempts to induce his patients to alter their diets. He complained to colleagues, "Changing a patient's diet is as difficult as changing his character structure!" The truth is, changing diet *is* changing character structure, or at least, the two must proceed together. As dietary habits are altered, related mental and emotional issues must be worked through, step by step.

Each change has the effect of disrupting one's modus operandi to some extent. If such changes are made very gradually, one is able to modify one's habits of behavior, thought, and emotion to correspond. The result can be a positive and gratifying evolution of the total person, supported by (though not totally a result of) dietary change.

But if dietary change is too abrupt, it won't "take," the necessary psychological adjustments cannot be managed. Then the effect is experienced as disturbing or even destructive. The diet becomes a "foreign body" in one's existence—a discordance that can be tolerated only to a point, and that then must be cast out and discontinued.

It is for this reason that many persons who attempt dietary improvement and move too quickly find themselves unable to adapt. They give up, go back to their prior diets, and conclude that the new diet just doesn't suit them. It has long been observed that those who make a successful transition to vegetarianism do it gradually, over a period of time. It's usually a stepwise process and seems most often to take place in several distinct stages.

Initially, there is the elimination of red meat. This commonly involves the gradual reduction of first beef and pork, and later other mammalian muscle meats such as veal and lamb. The next phase ordinarily entails the elimination of poultry. After that, fish and other seafoods may be reduced or eliminated, or they may be retained while the intake of dairy foods and eggs is lowered. Some people may take quite a long time in the first phase, others may

The Transition Plan

Phase	Eliminate
1.	red meat
2.	poultry
3.	fish or dairy

take many months or even years in the second and third. Those who have made the transition most successfully have remained at each phase until they felt comfortable with it and no longer felt that it was unnatural or that it was a strain.

This series of steps is not something artificial, imposed mechanically by physicians or nutritionists. Rather, it is a pattern that has frequently emerged in widely different settings and in very different people as a result of their own personal exploration and through their own processes of trial and error. It is tempting to wonder why it is that this particular sequence is so common. When one asks those who have followed it, they usually respond that they first eliminated what seemed to be most heavy and difficult to digest and caused the most problems. After adjusting to that, they then eliminated the food that seemed to be the next most objectionable.

Interestingly enough, the stepwise elimination of first red meat, then poultry, and finally fish corresponds to the elimination from the diet of the more evolved animals first. This is certainly a logical progression if one is becoming a vegetarian on a moral or ethical basis. The same pattern, however, has been observed in those people who wished to make the transition strictly for health reasons.

Replacing What's Dropped and Upgrading What's Not

But there is more to a successful transition than merely eliminating animal foods. At each step, as one category of foods is dropped other critical items should be added, so as both to maintain and improve the nutritional value of the diet. During Phase 1 the amount of sugar should be reduced; many people report that sugar increases the craving for meat, and vice versa. One should begin to experiment with combinations of grains and legumes. Taking legumes, such as lentils, garbanzos, or kidney beans, along with a grain is a basic principle in vegetarian nutrition. This is an element of the vegetarian diet that is so important that it should be progressively expanded and empha- sized as the transition proceeds.

During Phase 2, as poultry is eliminated, other refined foods, such as those based on white flour and those that are prepackaged, should be reduced. At this time fresh, cooked, green vegetables can become a focus, and one should make a consistent effort to have regular servings of them. The leafy greens, such as spinach, chard, or kale, are especially valuable. If fish is phased out, one might concentrate on reducing the fats and oils in the diet, while making sure that a reliable source of vitamin B_{12}, such as dairy products, is included on a regular basis. (See figure.)

The Transition Plan

Phase	Eliminate	Reduce	Add
1.	red meat	sugar	grains/legume combination
2.	poultry	refined foods	green (leafy) vegetables
3.	fish or dairy	fats and oils	dairy*

*As a source of B_{12}, supplementary protein, and trace elements, moderate but substantial and regular quantities of dairy products, eggs, or fermented soy products are used by most vegetarians. As an alternative, fish might be retained, with the result that eggs and dairy products are less needed. In later chapters, some of the pros and cons of these choices will be examined, along with the reasons why the use of dairy products might be considered the best choice.

This book is designed to lead one toward, and to prepare one for, a diet that is not merely vegetarian but is also solid, substantial, and sound. The principles presented here are based on some of the most ancient and respected traditional teachings on nutrition along with the most up-to-date research in the field. This combination has been tempered by many years of clinical experience with vegetarian diets in a modern setting.

Eliminating animal food does not automatically make the diet healthier. Rather, it provides the opportunity to make changes in the diet that can greatly improve health and well-being. But if these changes are not properly made, health and well-being can actually suffer due to the discontinuation of animal foods. Unfortunately the knowledge needed to make such changes often seems to be wanting. Indeed, it often appears that the popular vegetarian scene is ruled by chaos and confusion. There are many versions of vegetarianism, each with its adherents, who can be vocal or even evangelical in their fervor.

Unfortunately the scientific literature is, itself, far from crystal clear. While it may be overflowing with data about the negative effects of one food or the benefits of another, it provides scarcely a hint about how to organize all this information into a practical approach to eating.

In any case, it would seem prudent to equip the aspiring vegetarian with as much knowledge as possible about the ideal way to balance a nonmeat meal. In line with such a goal, this book is designed to provide the reader with both an understanding of relevant aspects of the science of nutrition and practical guidelines for food selection and preparation. Each chapter will include a discussion of the issues and the nutrients that are most important during that phase of the transition as well as suggestions for how to translate this information into menus and meals.

GETTING STARTED

Even before we begin to explore the issues surrounding meat in the next chapter, those readers who are interested in beginning the transition to vegetarianism can take a few preliminary steps. But before doing so, such persons might wish to get some perspective on where they're starting from.

At the outset, it is often helpful to survey one's overall diet so as to understand where one is beginning. Without a clear view of one's current habits, it is difficult to know what needs to be changed. This may be accomplished by a simple diet log. It's usually best to keep a record for at least four days of everything

Diet Record

8:00   *6 oz. freshly squeezed orange juice*

8:30   *one fried egg, 2 strips bacon, 2 pieces*
       buttered toast
       a cup of decaf coffee with milk and 1 tsp.
       sugar

10:30   *a cheese Danish*
        one cup coffee with cream and 1 tsp. sugar

12:30   *turkey on rye with lettuce, tomato and mayo,*
        one dill pickle, 1 small package corn chips,
        iced tea with lemon and 1 tsp. sugar

4:30   *an apple, 1 package roasted, salted peanuts,*
       and a diet cola

7:30   *tuna casserole, steamed fresh broccoli,*
       3 pieces Italian (white) bread, apple pie
       with ice cream
       a cup of decaf coffee

9:00   *8 oz. chocolate milk*
       ½ piece apple pie

11:00   *a diet soda*

A typical diet record of a better than average American diet. The diet could be significantly improved and brought under better control by eliminating the highlighted between-meal snacks.

eaten. This allows an objective viewing of the diet, and a number of improvements that can already be made will usually be immediately obvious. (See figure.)

Snacking

The most commonly needed change is simplification. Modern life presents continuous promptings to buy and consume an infinite variety of snacks and junk foods. These complicate the diet and confuse the palate so that one's sensitivity to one's needs is confounded. It's difficult to know when one is hungry and when one isn't, what one should eat and what one shouldn't. A first important step is to decrease or largely eliminate the nonnutrient items that pop out of vending machines and turn up beside cash registers. This will clear the air so that more serious issues of nutrition can come into evidence.

Revision of Eating Habits

1. Keep a diet log.
2. Reduce snacking.
3. Simplify meals.
4. Make all changes gradually.

The whole process of simplifying the diet and eliminating junk is greatly facilitated by limiting one's eating to three times a day. If food consumption is focused at three periods (meals), one can give it sufficient attention to regulate and refine it. Otherwise, habits acquired over many years will subvert all efforts to bring the diet under scrutiny or to improve it. Unconscious eating is the greatest pitfall in working with diet.

Even such changes as this will have powerful though subtle effects on one's mind and body. Like the elimination of animal foods, dietary modifications that involve phasing out extraneous items with little nutritional value should also be carried out gradually.

Breakfasts Without Meat

If one uses red meat frequently, one can prepare for the first phase of the transition by whittling down meat meals to one a day. A good place to start is with breakfasts. Breakfasts without meat are not difficult, and in fact offer much more opportunity for variety than the usual bacon, eggs, and toast.

The meat part of a breakfast is usually what is depended upon to give the texture and substance to the meal. When this is dropped out, the presence of more substantial nonmeat foods, like whole-grain cereals or the heavier whole-grain breads, become more

Here are some simple, commonly available, and easily prepared breakfast options.

Light Breakfast: Fruit-based

For example, have half a canteloupe or half a grapefruit. Or wait till midmorning and have 12 ounces of freshly squeezed orange or grapefruit juice. This will leave one hungry at about the right time for a noon lunch. Waiting is especially useful if dinner the night before was heavy or taken late.

Medium Breakfast: Add Grain

Have fruit or fruit juice first, then after a brief interval, grain and milk: for example, dry cereal with dairy or soy-based milk, or toast with cottage cheese, or nut butter or yogurt with cooked buckwheat cereal, etc.

Heavy Breakfast: More Protein

After the fruit or fruit juice, have, for instance, scrambled eggs in a whole-wheat pita, or scrambled tofu with toast and sub-acid fruit, or oatmeal cooked in milk topped with nut butter, or sautéed tofu.

interesting and appealing since they provide the taste, texture, and substance that came before from the meat.

Breakfast should be kept light unless one is physically active before lunch, or has eliminated the evening meal. In general you will find throughout the transition process that the progressive reduction of animal foods, processed foods, and very greasy and sweet foods will allow you to feel energetic and satisfied even though you're eating a reduced quantity of food overall.

With these few preliminary steps taken to reduce meat and to improve the overall quality of the diet, you are prepared to approach the subject of red meat in depth. The information in the next chapter will allow you to decide whether you wish to eliminate red meat completely from the diet and, if so, will allow you to implement those changes that help to replace what the meat offered nutritionally.

PHASE 1

RED MEAT

The first major step toward a vegetarian diet almost always involves the reduction or total elimination of red meat. Most often this means beef or pork. In a broader sense, red meat includes the flesh of all mammals—game animals such as deer or rabbits and the edible portions of livestock such as cows, pigs, calves, or sheep. The term is used more or less in contradistinction to fish and fowl, the flesh of which usually is not as red.

Man's consumption of meat dates back to his distant past when he still functioned almost exclusively as a hunter. The animals he ate were a part of an intact ecological system, as was man himself. This early ancestor of modern man had to adapt his digestion and metabolism to what was available, and so he evolved, learning to use the food at hand. Somewhat later, in the more recent past, man began to keep domestic animals for slaughter and consumption. Though this must have had some impact on the nature of the meat he ate, the changes were relatively minor. In recent years, however, major and far-reaching disruptions of the conditions under which such animals live have occurred. Advances in biology and technology have been harnessed to increase the ease and rapidity with which meat is produced, and while the results, in terms of productivity and price, have been gratifying, there has been a drastic alteration in the quality of meat that is commonly consumed.

This chapter will first review some of the fascinating (though at times grim) facts about the dangers of meat that are currently emerging. Along the way, it will detail techniques for minimizing or avoiding these dangers until meat can be gradually reduced and phased out of the diet. Then we will describe some of the ways to replace what is lost from the diet when meat is dropped, and how this can be done in a way that not only maintains the nutritional quality of the diet, but actually improves it.

Hormones in Meat

Probably the best-known problem with meat production relates to the use of diethylstilbestrol (DES). DES gained notoriety in the 1970s, when it was recognized as a cause of cancer in young women whose mothers had received it during pregnancy to prevent miscarriages. These "DES babies" and their difficulties made the drug a household word. DES is a synthetic compound that acts in the body as a female hormone, despite the fact that it is not found in nature.

Twenty years before the dangers of DES came to light, it had begun to be widely used as a feed additive. For reasons still not fully understood, it was found to promote growth in livestock. Since it was synthetic, it could be produced cheaply. DES increased weight gain by 15% to 19% in steers, which meant that for the relatively small cost of the minute amount of the drug required for a typical steer, the rancher might produce an extra 50 pounds of marketable meat. This was a great economic boon to cattle farmers.

One of the unusual properties of DES is that, unlike most natural hormones, it is readily absorbed through the digestive tract. This meant it could be added to animal feed, but it also means that it can be absorbed by the consumer who eats the meat of the animals raised on DES-supplemented feeds. When such meat is eaten, DES can enter one's body and be active. Only very small amounts are necessary to produce major effects. When DES was implanted in male chickens to "chemically castrate" them in the 1950s, men who had eaten them began to show signs of feminization, such as breast enlargement. Shortly thereafter the FDA stopped the use of DES for this purpose and was forced to purchase 10 million dollars' worth of contaminated poultry to get it off the market.[1]

At about the same time that adverse publicity about DES babies was bringing the drug to the attention of the public, residues of it were found in beef liver, and the FDA moved to stop its use in animal feeds. As a result, ranchers switched to another route of administration. DES pellets were implanted beneath the skin of the ear, a site where high concentrations of the drug would be least dangerous, since that part of the animal is usually not eaten but discarded after slaughter. From the implant site small amounts of the hormone are slowly absorbed into the body, where they stimulate growth. Though the implants themselves were not likely to find their way into the meat supply, the hormone was still present in small but significant amounts throughout the animal. In 1973 the FDA banned the use of implants. The livestock industry responded with legal proceedings and managed to overturn the ban. It was not until 1979 that the ruling was restored and the further sale and shipment of DES finally became illegal.

Nevertheless, it was discovered in 1980 that 50,000 head of cattle in Texas had been implanted with DES despite the reactivated ban. A subsequent probe revealed that such violations were widespread. At least 344,000 animals on 115 separate ranches in 16 different states had been illegally implanted. There was a considerable uproar over the matter, and most of the implants were removed from the steers, which were then held for a period of time to allow the dissipation of the drug before marketing. Though some cases of the illegal use of DES are still occasionally discovered, by and large its use seems to have been discontinued in the United States.

But the economic pressure to use such drugs is enormous. As a result, DES has now been replaced by a variety of similar hormones that have much the same effect on animal growth. At present, about 99% of all commercially raised feedlot cattle are treated with them. Synovex, which is the most popular of these, is implanted in the ear of the animal in the same fashion as was DES, and produces similar increases in weight gain. The 22 million cattle treated with it in 1983 yielded 185 million pounds of additional beef protein with no additional protein input.

Fortunately these new drugs seem to be safer than DES. In contrast to DES, they are naturally occurring hormones and are not readily absorbed from the intestinal tract. The dosages that reach the consumer seem to be harmless. It has been estimated that the amount of the drug taken in through treated beef would be only about one ten-thousandth of what the body itself produces. Unfortunately, however, other hormones are being used for different purposes, and their effects have not been explored as fully as have those of the growth promoters. For example, Melengestrol acetate (MGA), another synthetic female hormone (a progesterone), is used frequently as a feed additive to quiet heifers in heat. The use of this drug has aroused concern because it has been suspected of being a co-carcinogen, an agent which can act in concert with another to cause cancer.

Hormones constitute only one of the classes of substances found in meat that can be harmful. Pesticides have also gained a place of increasing importance in the farmer's chemical armamentarium. For example, insecticides are used to control the flies that swarm around livestock, biting the animals and causing them to become agitated and restless. Flies also interrupt their feeding and may spread disease. An agricultural report in 1979 estimated that animal losses suffered by the livestock and poultry industries as a result of flies amounted to around $4 billion annually.[2] Such an enormous economic toll must seem to the rancher to justify those risks he might incur in using toxic chemicals.

One of the most popular of the insecticides used to control flies in livestock lots is Vapona. It is an organophosphate similar to those used on field crops. Though not persistent in the environment, it is a nerve poison and included by the Environmental Protection Agency in the most highly toxic category of insecticides.

Yet cattle ranches routinely spray feedlots with it. As an

observer has noted, "It is not uncommon to see large tractor-driven sprayers equipped with banks of high pressure nozzles being driven down access roads, fogging pens, and sometimes the animals inside, with a cloud [of insecticide]. . . . In larger feedlots, where such application by tractor is time-consuming and often ineffective, managers sometimes turn to aerial spraying."[3] Another method is to "dip" livestock or create swim-through tanks filled with lindane, another organophosphate.

Though such insecticides generally do not persist into the final meat or animal products, the way they are used reflects the rather cavalier attitude of cattle ranchers toward chemicals that can be, and on a number of occasions have been, very harmful to those handling them. What emerges repeatedly from a survey of livestock management is this casual approach on the part of both ranchers and drug and feed suppliers to the multitude of drugs and chemicals they employ, some of which are very potent and potentially dangerous. The result is a pattern of overuse that leads not only to hazardous working conditions for cattlemen but to a habit of dependence on chemicals.

Though the hazards of individual substances are difficult to put into perspective or to evaluate, the overall picture is sobering. A report from the General Accounting Office maintained that 143 chemical residues are present in meat at levels above those set by the government as tolerable. Of these, 42 are thought to be cancer-causing and 26 have been associated with birth defects and fetal mutations.[4] The additive effects of such a confusing conglomeration of chemicals is a research challenge of some magnitude. Moreover, the constant use of hormones to increase growth, insecticides to control pests, and a wide range of drugs and medications (to subdue and suppress the diseases that arise in less than healthy animals) has made it increasingly possible to market livestock that is sickly and substandard.

Meat Inspection

Hogs are known to collapse sometimes on the loading docks of slaughterhouses, and the carcasses of steers are sometimes found to have cancer. "If the tumor is benign, we will pass it," says one meat inspector, "but if it is malignant and has spread, out it goes." But some slaughterhouses find it impossible to pass up the hefty profit to be made by purchasing sick animals. "They buy junk cows at ten cents a pound and sell them at ten times that amount. . . . They can afford to have a few carcasses condemned."[5] Unfortunately, meat inspectors can catch only a small fraction of the violations. Their approach is to monitor—that is, to make a random sampling of carcasses for disease and chemical residues. They cannot possibly evaluate in any thorough way each animal that is slaughtered. Usually the meat has gone to the stores and has been eaten by the time the tests come back from the lab. Test results that show dangerous residues or disease then tip the inspectors off to examine more carefully animals from that particular source next time, and allow them to identify those suppliers who regularly send through sick and contaminated animals.

But the inspector's job is difficult; he works in the slaughterhouse alongside its employees and management, and inevitably comes under pressure not to find too many violations. To do so would jeopardize the business and the jobs of his friends.

Official agencies have reported a high incidence of inadequate inspection and have made recommendations for improvements, but such corrections have not been forthcoming. There are difficulties of impressive proportions, both with infected meat and with chemical residues. The FDA recently stated that of the 600 chemical residues present in our meat supply, only 10% are regularly monitored by government agencies.[6]

The situation with hygiene is equally disturbing. In 1983 it was discovered that a large meatpacker in Colorado with a $20 million contract to supply school cafeterias had been slaughtering diseased and dead cattle, some of which were infected with salmonella. The next year a meatpacking concern and a pet food company in Pennsylvania were indicted for a conspiracy to buy dead and dying animals purportedly for use in pet food, only to resell them to outlets that supplied hospitals and schools.[7]

Parasites in Meat

Animal foods also carry the risk of transmitting parasites. In contrast to those microbes such as bacteria that are technically plantlife, parasites are members of the animal kingdom. They range from one-celled protozoa to more complex multi-celled forms of life, the most common being worm-like animals. Although a variety of parasites plague livestock and can enter the human body from infected meat, as far as we now know only two are presently causing widespread and serious disease in the United States.

The first of these parasites is that which produces toxo-plasmosis. Up to 40% of the adult population in this country has antibodies to *Toxoplasma gondii,* reflecting some degree of infection at some point in life. Although most cases are mild enough to escape diagnosis, it is estimated that 40% of the infants born to women who become actively infected while pregnant may develop clinical disease. Experts say that in the U.S. alone, more than 3,000 infants are born each year to such mothers, and that, of these, about 1 out of 10 will die, 1 of 5 will suffer blindness or brain damage, and approximately two thirds of those who seem normal will later develop active infections. Though toxoplasmosis has long been known to cause blindness and retardation in newborns, its prevalence was not fully appreciated until recently.[nt.1]

In the United States, pigs are probably the most common carrier of the disease, but one phase of the parasite's life cycle also takes place in the household cat. Though many infections are acquired from meat, direct infection from cats is probably also common.

A number of cases have been reported in those eating uncooked or lightly cooked hamburger, though it is possible that the infection came from pork or mutton, since ground beef is often stretched with odds and ends of other meats. In any case, experts feel that livestock is probably so widely infected that the emphasis of preventive programs should be on cooking meat thoroughly and handling it carefully so that the parasites can't be transmitted to food from raw meat by means of tables, utensils, cutting boards, and so on.[8]

Trichinosis is the other widespread parasitic infestation acquired by eating meat. Again, it is a disease that is acquired from pork and one that has long been known, but one that has only recently been discovered to be more common than previously thought. The U.S. has one of the world's highest rates of *T. spiralis* infection among both humans and animals, and authorities say that the disease is an important public health problem. The prevalence of the infection is reflected by the fact that autopsy sampling of muscle tissue from the human diaphragm alone found infection in 2.2% of the population, and this sort of test picks up only a fraction of those affected. Experts feel that many cases are misdiagnosed, since the symptoms are not specific to this disease. They include such common complaints as loss of appetite, abdominal cramps, and diarrhea. Muscle and joint pains, low-grade fever, and skin eruptions may develop as the larvae penetrate the muscles and other tissues. Such ailments are likely to be misdiagnosed as arthritis, influenza, or dermatitis. Symptoms may continue for months or years, until the larvae are encapsulated and calcified. Though most people with trichinosis recover, some develop chronic heart disease.[8]

It appears that the incidence of trichinosis has decreased somewhat since the advent of regulations requiring the cooking of the garbage that is used for hog food, since that was a major route of reinfection. But there are presently no tests or inspections of pork in slaughterhouses to detect *T. spiralis*. Though such inspection is practiced in Europe and has been highly successful, it was discontinued in the U.S. in 1906. For this reason the thorough cooking of all pork products is important to prevent infection.

The Meat Market

Though the meat coming from the slaughterhouses may be of questionable quality, what happens to it in the retail stores is even more disturbing. Although federal inspectors are stationed in slaughterhouses, the surveillance of supermarkets is left to state and local officials, who may make visits only at infrequent intervals. Economic pressures in the retail store often lead to faster, slipshod, work and shortcuts in the cleaning of equipment and facilities. Bad conditions commonly result.[9]

The floors of the cutting, storage, and packaging areas build up layers of grease, blood, and decomposing meat, and provide a tempting place for bacteria to grow. Meat delivered on loading docks may sit for some time before being unpacked and stored, despite the fact that even brief periods of warmer temperatures can result in accelerated spoilage. In some cases, slimy and outdated meats are unwrapped, scrubbed down, and repackaged.[10] This is especially dangerous in the case of ham, which may be sliced and served with no further cooking, or with such meats as ground beef or hot dogs, which may not be cooked thoroughly. Over 40% of a sampling of frankfurters had more than enough bacteria growing in them to consider them "spoiled" by accepted standards.[11]

Some of the bacteria growing in spoiled foods can cause disease. Salmonella is one that is a common cause of what we often call "food poisoning," and infections with it seem to be on the increase. In the United States, diagnosed cases recently reached 44,000 per year, approximately four times as many as 20 years earlier.[12] Infections with salmonella affect particularly the gastro-intestinal tract, producing diarrhea, abdominal pain, and a disordered digestion. In the past, such food poisoning was not considered a serious illness, for it was rarely life-threatening. If the symptoms became severe, it could be cleared up quickly with a short course of antibiotics.

But recently the whole issue of salmonella infection has taken a dark and ominous turn. Cases are beginning to turn up, traceable to infected meat, that do not respond to treatment with ordinary antibiotics. They are drug-resistant, and as a result, people who have developed the infection have died with increasing frequency.[13] What's more, this is only the tip of the iceberg. Such meat-borne infections have grave and far-reaching implications for the health of the public. To understand the seriousness and the magnitude of this problem, we must explore briefly the use of antibiotics in animal feeds.

Antibiotic-Resistant Microbes

The first antibiotics used in modern medicine were the sulfa drugs, discovered in the 1930s. These were followed in 1941 by the discovery of penicillin and then, within a few years, by a number of others, including tetracycline. As early as 1949 researchers at one of the large pharmaceutical houses noticed that animals given a mash containing residues of tetracycline gained 10% to 20% more weight than normal. Why this is true is still not well understood, though it appears that the effect may be particularly prominent where animals suffer from the stress that comes with crowded conditions. In any case, as a result of using small doses of an antibiotic like tetracycline in the food supply, it became possible to raise animals in less space, producing more meat with the same amount of feed. The effect is similar to that produced by hormones.

In the U.S. today some nine million tons of antibiotics per year go into animal feed as a growth promoter,[14] an amount at least equal to all the antibiotics used to treat infections in humans and animals. Such widespread use has led to some concern about the presence of antibiotics in the diet, since some people who are allergic to them may have reactions to meat that is contaminated. Although this may, in fact, be a minor problem, a much more serious complication is that of antibiotic resistance.

Antibiotics were not invented by man. In fact, their existence goes way back in the history of life on this planet—for antibiotics are part of the repertoire of weapons that microorganisms use to compete with one another. It is said that Sir Alexander Fleming discovered penicillin when he left a culture plate sitting on the windowsill of his laboratory. There was a conspicuous bare spot in the midst of the growth of bacteria that he had planted in the plate; a mold was growing in the center of the clear space and had apparently produced some substance that killed the bacteria surrounding it. Now we know that this was not an isolated phenomenon, but that all fungi have the capacity to manufacture such antibiotic substances.

They developed such a capacity long ago, as a result of their being so often in competition with bacteria for space and nourishment. The two basic microorganisms that live in the soil are fungi and bacteria. Many fungi feed on the same dead plant material that bacteria grow in, setting the two classes of microbes at odds. Thus crowded by bacteria, the fungi have developed the ability to elaborate poisons and keep them at bay.

But bacteria are not without defenses of their own. They developed a mechanism by means of which they could resist fungal antibiotics and not be affected by them. This capacity for antibiotic resistance is part of the basic nature of bacteria, though microbiologists have only recently begun to understand the complexity and efficiency of the process.

More than Darwinian Selection

Until recently it was felt that though antibiotic resistance was a problem, it was a manageable one, because by the time resistant infections appeared, we would already have developed new antibiotics to which the new microbes were not yet resistant. But as it turns out, we have grossly underestimated the humble bacterium. Its resistance to antibiotics is not a mere process of Darwinian selection, it's an active adaptation. Though only a one-celled organism, it has the capacity, no doubt developed during millennia of struggle against fungi, to recognize antibiotics and produce small gene-like particles that alter its metabolism so that it is unaffected by the antibiotic. This seems to be what occurs in the intestinal tracts of farm animals and results in antibiotic-resistant microbes.

Now, this wouldn't matter so much if it weren't for the fact that the intestinal tracts of farm animals carry some bacteria that cause disease in humans. The best-known example of this is salmonella. Foods made with meat that has even small numbers of these bacteria remaining on it spoil easily. The spoilage involves the growth of the bacteria, and the food then has the capacity to cause food poisoning.

But antibiotic-resistant strains of salmonella are becoming increasingly more common and as a result salmonella food poisoning is progressively more difficult to treat. A recent report by the Center for Disease Control found that while only 0.2% of cases of ordinary salmonellosis resulted in death, 4.2% of those caused by resistant strains were fatal.[15] Two thirds of those infections could be traced to livestock.[nt.2]

Moreover, the bad news doesn't end there. It appears that microbes have the capacity, when exposed to constant antibiotic dosages, to develop resistance to other antibiotics that they've never been exposed to. When pigs were fed trace amounts of tylosin, a new antibiotic, resistance to erythromycin and other antibiotics appeared on the particles that carry resistance.[17-19] Though most animals are fed only a single antibiotic as a growth promoter, a study done in 1984 found multiple drug resistances in 80% of 3,500 cultures of salmonella made from livestock.[20]

Communicating Resistance

Unfortunately, this is still only a small part of the story. As our understanding of antibiotic resistance has become more sophisticated, we have learned that resistance-carrying particles need not be developed by every microbe. Rather, they can be exchanged between microbes and then passed on to succeeding generations. This explains why resistance to antibiotics can arise so quickly and spread so rapidly. Moreover—what's even more amazing and of even graver import—such particles can be transferred between microbes of different species. For instance, a harmless bacterium from the intestinal tract can transfer its antibiotic resistance to a different, more virulent microbe. The implications of this have caused serious concern among scientists. Resistant germs, developed as a matter of course in the intestinal tracts of animals or humans that have been given antibiotics, can pass on that resistance to microbes that cause such diseases as meningitis, or syphilis, and then those diseases can no longer be treated successfully with previously used antibiotics. In fact, such a process may well account for the increasing number of cases of drug-resistant infections, and the increasing mortality from such previously easily treatable infectious diseases as pneumonia.

The picture that emerges is nothing short of mind-boggling. At any given moment, a half *billion* animals are being fed the continuous small doses of antibiotics that produce microbes with multiple antibiotic resistances. These resistant germs are being released into the environment primarily through meat products. They have not only the (relatively minor) ability to cause disease themselves, but also the potential capacity to pass their drug resistances on to the microbes that cause our most serious infectious diseases.[19]

A Storm on the Horizon

Such issues can be truly explosive for the meat industry. A recent news special by NBC observed that cases of food poisoning from antibiotic-resistant salmonella in California had more than tripled in the preceding year. State health officials believed that a major route of infection was contaminated hamburger. At the same time that infection rates with the resistant salmonella were climbing, the Department of Agriculture had begun an extensive investigation of meatpacking plants. It "turned up evidence that at least 14 percent of the plants were producing adulterated, contaminated meat."[21] The Agriculture Department's report on meatpacking conditions, which would create shock waves around the country if its implications for the rising incidence of resistant infections were fully understood, had been written by middle-level officials, but had then mysteriously disappeared, according to the investigating reporter.

Health officials in California confirm that the incidence of drug-resistant salmonella infection rose at an alarming rate in the year 1985, and that preliminary figures for 1986 showed a continuing increase. What's more, fatalities are being reported with disturbing frequency.[22] Persons recently taking antibiotics for other reasons seem particularly susceptible to severe food poisoning of this type.[23] Apparently the antibiotic, by wiping out the normal population of bacteria in the intestine, makes it more susceptible to the rapid growth of salmonella.

Such an ominous picture is far from appealing, and it is

not surprising that there is resistance from many quarters to dealing with it openly. But until there is greater awareness of the magnitude of the problem, there will continue to be serious risks to the public health. In the meantime, those who are well informed will take careful precautions.

In fact, in the face of such overwhelming facts about the meat supply, one might feel compelled to stop eating all red meat immediately. But as discussed in the first chapter, abrupt dietary change is rarely advisable or successful. If one is accustomed to taking large amounts of meat, the best approach is to reduce it gradually. While one is reducing the amount of red meat, one can ensure one's safety by taking care to handle the meat cautiously.

What to Do: The Prudent Use of Meat

The danger comes from raw meat; once meat is cooked thoroughly it is safe. Rare or undercooked meat may spread infection,[24] as may (barely) adequately cooked meat or meat dishes, especially if they are allowed to sit for long periods while warm. Bacteria like salmonella do not grow at all during refrigeration, nor do they grow significantly at normal room temperature. But they don't die at those temperatures either, and may remain for weeks to cause infection. Therefore surfaces that are in contact with raw meats must be cleaned carefully. The following rules to minimize the risk of infection from antibiotic-resistant microbes represent a consensus of opinion by current health officials:[12]

1. Don't put leaky packages of raw meat on the upper shelves of the refrigerator or on top of a loaded grocery cart, where they can drip on other foods, especially those that won't be cooked.
2. Don't use the same counters or cutting boards for vegetables and raw meat unless vegetables are to be cooked. Surfaces on which raw meat is handled should be washed carefully before other uses.
3. All utensils used for meat as well as sponges or cloths used for cleaning should go into hot sudsy water.
4. Hands should be washed thoroughly after handling raw meat.

5. Meat should be well cooked. It should not be held at room temperature for long periods afterward, but should be cooled rapidly and then refrigerated.
6. Cooked meat and meat dishes should be reheated thoroughly before serving again.

MEATS AND FATS: THE IMPACT ON HEALTH

To say that methods of raising livestock and of handling meat have undermined the health of the animals and the value of meat products will now seem like a quiet understatement. Risks from chemicals, drugs, parasites, and especially exposure to resistant microbes provide ample reason to begin to phase out meat. But what if one could obtain meat from healthy animals grown under ideal conditions—meat of good quality, with no drug residues, that had been handled carefully? What if one's supermarket began to offer (as some now do) meat from animals raised with no drugs, chemicals, or growth promoters? How would meat stack up then as a dietary staple?

It certainly has some nutritional strengths. It is high in protein and provides a rich supply of certain minerals, most notably iron. It is also a reliable source of some vitamins, especially vitamin B_{12}. But it is almost totally lacking in other vitamins, such as C, E, and folic acid, and is a very poor source of other important minerals, such as calcium. Moreover, even the absence of drugs, chemicals, and growth-promoting antibiotics doesn't ensure freedom from parasites like toxoplasma or trichinella. But perhaps the most serious drawback to meat is its fat content.

Meat at its very best is moderate to high in fat, and the amount of fat that comes along with a protein meal is very important. If one automatically takes in large amounts of fat in the process of getting the protein one needs, fat levels can easily become excessive—one of the major criticisms of the American diet is its unusually high content of fat. The average American takes in 40% to 45% of his calories as fats and oils. Besides making for one of the greasiest diets in the world, such fat levels increase one's risk of some of the more serious health problems.

Percentage of Protein, Fat, and Carbohydrate Calories in Meats

Food (Uncooked)	Protein (% of calories)	Fat (% of calories)	Carbo- hydrate (% of calories)
Steak, T-bone, 62% lean, 38% fat	15%	85%	0.0%
Steak,,flank, 100% lean	60%	40%	0.0%
Ham, retail cuts, medium fat	20%	80%	0.0%
Hamburger, regular ground	30%	70%	0.0%
Lamb, composite of cuts, medium fat	25%	75%	0.0%
Chicken, roasters, flesh and skin	40%	60%	0.0%
Turkey, medium fat, flesh and skin	45%	55%	0.0%

Source: Watt & Merrill: *Handbook of the Nutritional Contents of Foods.*[25]

Dietary Fat and Cancer

In the previous chapter we saw that a vegetarian diet was associated with a decreased risk of cancer. Much of this protective effect probably stems from the fact that vegetarian diets are generally lower in fat than meat diets.[26,27] The evidence linking a high-fat diet with an increased incidence of cancer is now sufficient to justify significant changes in the American diet. Both individual researchers and a panel assembled by the National Academy of Sciences have recommended a substantial decrease in dietary fats and oils.[28,29] The connection between excessive fats and oils in the diet and malignancy is particularly well-established in the case of colon cancer, which accounts for 3% of all deaths (50,000 people per year) in the U.S. It has been estimated that 90% of the deaths from colon cancer in the U.S. could be eliminated by dietary modifications.[30] Research has consistently shown that a high-fat, low-fiber diet increases one's risk of developing this disease.[31-35]

Currently researchers talk of interactions of a variety of cancer-causing agents working in successive phases to produce a tumor. They speak of an initiation phase, during which a chemical irritant acts on cells, and a promotional phase, during which the malignancy proceeds to develop. Fats and oils are thought to act in concert with radiation or with environmental chemicals such as tars, drugs, or food additives to produce cancer.

One important co-carcinogen for chemical irritants acting on the lining of the colon is produced by certain bacteria living in the colon when they break down bile acids. Persons on a high-fat diet have more of these breakdown products, possibly because such persons require more bile to emulsify the larger amounts of fats and oils they've eaten. Although these substances have been found to have a promoting effect in the development of colon cancer, they cannot alone produce tumors. Our environments and diets contain countless substances, both naturally occurring and synthetic, that have been found to have the potential to independently initiate malignant growths, but we do not ordinarily ingest large enough quantities of them to create a serious problem. Nevertheless, it is possible that low levels of a number of them in the colon in the presence of a high concentration of a promoting agent can result in cancer.

It seems clear, then, why people on low-fat diets would have less colon cancer. But why would those on high-fiber diets also be protected? The explanation seems to lie in the fact that certain of the indigestible components of fruits, vegetables, grains, and beans provide the protective effect. Just as some of them carry chemical residues from the food out of the body through the feces, others have the capacity to pick up the altered bile acids, preventing them from acting on the intestinal lining. Thus dietary fiber can help in two ways. While some components may absorb bile acid residues that might promote tumor formation, others pick up the chemical compounds that would otherwise initiate the cancer.

Although researchers are in agreement on the benefits of high-fiber and low-fat diets, there are other points that are more controversial. For example, some studies have found a specific correlation between beef consumption and cancer of the colon.[36] When the beef consumption of different populations was compared with their incidence of large bowel cancer, a positive correlation of more than 0.9 was found (1.0 is a perfect correlation).[37] How the consumption of beef in particular might interplay with the action of bile acids and other carcinogens is not certain. In any case, it is clear that a well-balanced vegetarian diet, which is free of meat and tends to be low in fat and high in fiber, is good insurance against colon cancer.

High fat levels have also been found to be associated with some other cancers, most clearly with cancers of the breast and prostate. For example, research has shown that raising the total fat and oil content of the diet increases breast tumors in mice and rats.[38] A large number of separate studies comparing populations in different parts of the world have shown a higher incidence of breast cancer in those whose diets contain more fats and oils.[39-45]

Although it is thought that dietary fat has its own direct promoting effect on breast cancer, it may also increase one's risk of the disease indirectly by elevating hormone levels in women.[46] Vegetarian women excrete more estrogen and as a result have more moderate estrogen levels than do women who eat meat. It seems likely that the lower fat content of the vegetarian diet is responsible. Elevated estrogen levels are thought to be dangerous, since estrogen seems to play a facilitating role in the formation of breast cancer.[47]

Though lowering female hormone levels through a low-fat diet might sound as though it could undermine one's sexuality, the truth is that the extremely high-fat diet typical today in the U.S. has raised estrogen levels to abnormal heights. Elevated hormone levels are not only without value, they may also carry certain liabilities. High levels may not only predispose one to cancer of the breast, but also magnify the normal hormonal shifts that occur at menopause or even at menstruation. Premenstrual syndrome, with its irritability, fluid retention, depression, and tiredness, is thought by some researchers to be due in part to exaggerated estrogen levels, which reach their peak just prior to the onset of the menses. Taking progesterone, which counters the estrogen, has been helpful for some women. But it is not without serious side effects, and it would seem much preferable to reduce the elevated estrogen levels by shifting to a low-fat diet. Exercise and the loss of excess weight can also help to normalize estrogen levels.

The American diet is remarkable for its exaggerated content of fat. America is also noted for a preoccupation with sexual matters and for other rather unusual phenomena such as an exceptionally early onset of sexual maturity and menstruation in its young women. The discovery that a high-fat diet elevates hormone levels in women is fascinating and raises some interesting questions about the relationship between diet and the psychophysiology of sexuality. Could a transition to vegetarianism, if it were to occur on a large scale, have a subtle but significantly positive impact on the psychosocial fabric of our society?

Fat and Vascular Disease

Any diet designed to decrease fat should limit not only beef but also pork, since the latter is exceptionally high in fat. Moreover, clinicians have suspected a connection between pork consumption and hypertension. While this has not been investigated statistically, it has long been accepted by some experts in the field.[48] There is also research showing that even moderate beef consumption will produce a small but significant rise in blood pressure,[49] though not one so dramatic as that attributed to pork. Not only does hypertension (high blood pressure) contribute to the development of heart disease, as we saw in the last chapter, it also increases susceptibility to strokes, another major cause of death. Most of such vascular diseases are based on the same underlying process: atherosclerosis.

Atherosclerosis, or hardening of the arteries, involves deposition of a fatty substance in the linings of the blood vessels. The vessels affected gradually become clogged to the point that blood can't pass through. Ultimately tissues and organs deprived of an adequate blood supply will suffer damage. Either they deteriorate gradually, which we may interpret as premature aging, or else they die suddenly, producing the catastrophic events that we call heart attacks and strokes. Atherosclerosis is a disease that must concern all people in the modern industrialized societies because it is so common.

In the U.S. today, atherosclerotic diseases are the number one killer, responsible for over half of all the deaths that occur each year. Formerly considered a disease of older people, atherosclerosis seems to be attacking younger and younger people. A recent study of 35 youths ranging in age from 7 to 24 who had died of various causes found the early signs of atherosclerosis in all of them. The extent of the disease varied but was minimal only in the youngest. Since it is the arteries that are obstructed by atherosclerosis, the disease process affects all parts of the body, but the heart and brain (which need a continuous supply of blood) are most seriously threatened. In the above study early involvement of the coronary arteries was seen in all but 6 of the young people.[50]

Atherosclerotic diseases are, in fact, so pervasive that we have come to resign ourselves to them. Physicians now routinely accept evidence of atherosclerosis that is advancing with age as "normal." Yet if we could regain our objectivity on the subject, we would be forced to conclude that the affluent nations of the world are caught up in an epidemic of massive proportions. Approximately three of every five people will die of atherosclerosis and its resulting diseases. Yet the average person is aware of its existence only in the vaguest fashion. Connections in his mind between the details of how he lives and the development of disease are far from clear. The loss of objectivity here is all the more disturbing because current research suggests that the development of atherosclerosis could be significantly retarded, or even totally prevented, by a marked reduction in dietary fats and oils. Indeed, in countries such as Japan, when the population of certain regions took in less than 10% of their calories as fat (about one fourth the level consumed by Americans), atherosclerosis was virtually unknown.[51] Though clearly other factors contribute to the origin of such a disease, it is tempting to surmise that the low fat and oil intake is at least partly responsible for the low incidence of atherosclerosis. In fact, a number of scientific studies support this conclusion.[52]

Those who don't want anyone tampering with their eating habits will often say: "The most important thing you can do to prevent heart disease is to choose the right grandparents." Though it is clear that genetic predisposition plays some part in the development of atherosclerosis, this doesn't mean diet isn't important, too. Our genes provide a map of the diseases that we can develop *when* and *if* health deteriorates and our habits permit. We don't have to realize that particular negative potential. On the contrary, it is possible to lead an active healthy life and die without evident disease. In healthy populations, it is not uncommon to expire quietly in one's sleep at an advanced age, without ever suffering chronic illness or disability. Recent research has shown that even men with a genetically determined tendency to early, fatal, heart disease can, through a low-fat diet, reduce their serum cholesterol levels dramatically. This suggests that they can, like their grandfathers who had similar genes but healthy diets, live to a ripe old age rather than dying at the current average age of 45.[53]

Curing Coronary Heart Disease with Diet?

For the vast majority of us who have already developed a significant degree of atherosclerosis, there is even more exciting news. Recent research has shown that with proper dietary change there exists the possibility of reversing this serious condition. Only a few decades ago such ideas were dismissed out of hand. It was assumed that the deposits and damage of atherosclerosis, once they had taken place, were permanent. Now it has been conclusively demonstrated that this is not true. More sophisticated diagnostic tools and more rigorous diets have allowed us to document clearly the gradual disappearance of the plaques from the arterial walls.[54,55] It is, however, nearly impossible to design a healthful diet that will accomplish such a reversal without its being largely vegetarian.

The Pritikin diet is a case in point. Atherosclerosis has been treated with this diet, which eliminates all red meat, poultry, nuts, and seeds in order to reach an overall fat and oil content of close to 10% of total caloric intake. Results have been encouraging, but the idea is hardly new. Actually, a low-fat, low-protein rice diet was shown as early as 1947, by Walter Kempner at Duke University, to result in dramatic reversals of arterial disease.

Dr. Kempner was able, by maintaining patients with advanced

arterial disease on a diet of mostly rice for a minimum of six months (sometimes as much as several years), to produce dramatic improvements.[55] That significant changes had occurred in the arteries was suggested by the clearing seen on retinal exams of the patients treated. The one spot where a sampling of the blood vessels can be directly examined is in the eye. By using an ophthalmoscope, the physician can look at the small arteries and veins that stretch across the surface of the retina. These vessels are often taken to represent, with a fair degree of accuracy, the condition of the vascular system in general. Kempner took special photographs of these retinal vessels, showing their clogging with atherosclerotic plaque and the resulting damage, including hemorrhages, fatty deposits, and scars that could be seen on the surface of the retina. Some of the follow-up photographs in those patients who responded best showed completely normal, healthy retinae and retinal vessels. Such results were so out of keeping with current assumptions about the irreversibility of atherosclerosis that Kempner's colleagues were baffled. When he reported that the changes were produced by diet (along with a moderate amount of exercise), his case reports and photographs were not only ignored but sometimes ridiculed, and the implications of his work were overlooked for decades.

There is also some evidence that not only the fat but also the protein from animal sources may play an important role in the origin of atherosclerosis in experimental animals.[56,57] The same may be true for humans. Researchers in New Orleans studied the diets of deceased human subjects in relation to the degree of atherosclerotic plaque found in their coronary arteries on autopsy. Several factors seemed to be associated with less clogging of the arteries. One was increased complex carbohydrate, another was an increased proportion of vegetable protein in relation to animal protein.[58] Both these characteristics, of course, are most pronounced in a vegetarian diet. In fact, the researchers eventually realized (as anyone living in New Orleans should) that more complex carbohydrate and more vegetable protein could add up to only one thing: red beans and rice.[59] This is a favorite staple in the city of Mardi Gras, and tradition has it that a young man will never propose to a young lady until he's sampled her red beans and rice. This dish is the same as those that form the basis of many, if not most, ethnic diets that are largely vegetarian; that is, it features a combination of a grain and a legume.

The term "legume" is an important one for the aspiring vegetarian to comprehend. It does not, as the French word *legumes* suggests, mean any number of vegetables. A more familiar equivalent might be "beans and peas," but that's a bit ambiguous since "beans" can mean string beans, which are eaten before their leguminous seeds develop enough to have the nutritional properties of the beans and peas that are referred to here as legumes. One might try "peas and dried beans," but that leaves out fresh shelled beans, such as lima beans, which are both nutritious and more appealing than their dried equivalents. So it appears as though "legume," academic though it may seem, is here to stay. In any event, the important point is that legumes combine with grains to provide a good-quality vegetable protein. They also contain, as do grains, large quantities of complex carbohydrate.

CARBOHYDRATE: THE IDEAL FUEL

Since the use of protein is mainly for repair and replacement of the structural components of tissue, one needs smaller quantities of it than of those nutrients whose major use is as a source of energy. In the following chapter we will explore in detail the issue of exactly how much protein is needed, but for the moment our focus is on the question of fuel and energy needs. When one gets his protein from mostly vegetable sources instead of animal ones, his principal source of fuel automatically changes. Whereas with an animal-protein diet the major source of fuel is fat, with a diet in which protein comes from vegetable sources, the major source of fuel is carbohydrate.

This is inevitable; it is impossible to get vegetable protein without a generous amount of carbohydrate accompanying it, as we can see from the figure on the next page. Many people, foremost among them those who have suffered through popular weight-loss diets, may regard carbohydrate as anathema. If they

Percentage of Protein, Fat, and Carbohydrate Calories in Foods[nt.3]

Food (Uncooked)	Protein (% in calories)	Fat (% in calories)	Carbo- hydrate (% in calories)
Hamburger, regular ground	30%	70%	0.0%
Chicken, roasters, flesh and skin	40%	60%	0.0%
Rice	10%	5%	85%
Mung beans	25%	5%	70%
Spinach	40%	10%	50%
Broccoli	35%	5%	60%
Whole-wheat bread	15%	10%	75%
Yogurt, low fat	30%	30%	40%
Apple	1%	4%	95%
Almonds	10%	75%	15%

Source: Watt & Merrill: *Handbook of the Nutritional Contents of Foods.*[25]

hear that a vegetarian diet means more carbohydrate, then they are likely to recoil and dismiss it out of hand. But replacing fat with carbohydrate is hardly a disaster, since carbohydrate is vastly superior to fat as a fuel.

For, first of all, as a fuel carbohydrate "burns clean." Foods such as fat and carbohydrate are oxidized to supply energy for the functioning of the body. When their burning is finished, the waste from this process must be removed. The oxidation of carbohydrate is very straightforward: it yields only carbon dioxide and water. The carbon dioxide exits through the lungs, and the water through perspiration, urine, or the moisture of exhaled air. The metabolism of fat, however, is a different matter: not all of the fat molecule can be reduced to carbon dioxide and water; there are residues of acids and something called "the ketone body" that remain. Such noncombustible wastes are troublesome, creating acidity and disrupting normal metabolic activities.

Although only a limited amount of protein is necessary for structural repair, when meat is a major part of the diet it will often end up supplying more protein than is actually needed. The rest is burned as fuel, along with the fat of the meat. Such protein, like fat, also leaves a potentially troublesome residue of acid, as well as ammonia. Small to moderate amounts of such by-products are handled easily by the body, but when they become excessive they can be irritating. Though at one time an overgenerous supply of protein was considered an enviable luxury, in recent years ideas have begun to change. High-protein diets are now thought to cause progressive damage to the kidneys,[60] in part because of the residues that result. With this in mind, it becomes appropriate to limit protein intake to the range that is needed for tissue rebuilding and repair, and to avoid taking substantial amounts beyond that, which would end up being burnt as fuel.

A certain amount of energy-producing food is necessary each day. As mentioned previously, the average adult will need somewhere between 1,800 and 2,500 calories.[61] If we are to avoid fat and protein as major sources of fuel, then we are left with carbohydrate as the only other possibility. This is quite as it should be, since carbohydrate might be considered the ideal fuel. Nature takes carbon dioxide and water and puts them together in the presence of light, a process we call photosynthesis. Thus is captured the energy of the sun. We crack open the package, remove the energy, and cast off the carbon dioxide and water, which our bodies are designed to handle quite comfortably.

Carbohydrates: The Good and the Bad

But not all carbohydrate is the same. There are two basic types: simple and complex. Simple carbohydrate is sugar, and there are many different types of sugars—sucrose, fructose, and glucose, for example. Sugar molecules are relatively small. They might be considered the basic carbohydrate units. Since complex carbo-hydrates are much larger molecules composed of countless sugar units in long chains, they are broken down gradually, releasing the sugar links one by one into the bloodstream. The sugar units themselves, if taken into the body alone in any substantial quantity, will flood the circulation, playing havoc with blood sugar levels and causing physiological and emotional instability.

A sudden rise in blood sugar also requires a sudden output of insulin, since insulin is required for glucose to pass from the bloodstream into the cells. Frequent high doses of concentrated sugar thus put a strain on the insulin-producing cells of the pancreas, perhaps eventually disabling them and interfering with their capacity to smoothly regulate blood sugar levels. Such disorders as "hypoglycemia" and eventually even diabetes[62] may follow. For such reasons, complex carbohydrate is much preferable to the simple form as a major constituent of the diet. The principal complex carbohydrate in the diet is starch.

It's unfortunate that starch has gotten such bad press. The habitual dieter might inform his physician with an air of smug pride, "I avoid starchy foods almost entirely." Yet from the point of view of good health, starch should constitute the bulk of the well-balanced diet, since it's the best fuel. Fuel needs exceed other needs, so starch should supply the major portion of the calories one consumes.

But starch, too, comes in a variety of forms. Some starchy foods, such as white bread, are very low in nutrients other than calories. Although starch is a better fuel than sugar, fat, or protein, it is much more desirable to get starch from whole grains, vegetables, legumes, and fruits, where it is accompanied by some quantity of vitamins and minerals, protein, and fiber. The fiber in whole, starchy plant foods, for example, has been shown to further slow the absorption of sugar units from the starch chain into the circulation.[63,64] Thus starch in the form of vegetables, grains, and beans is especially unlikely to throw blood sugar levels out of kilter. Vitamins and minerals are also important. Just as one can't burn gasoline in an automobile engine without spark plugs and piston rings, carbohydrate can't be oxidized without the metabolic machinery that requires vitamins and minerals. But, like engine parts, cellular components wear out and must be regularly replaced. Without an ongoing supply of the vitamins and minerals and proteins needed for their manufacture, one cannot keep the metabolic machinery in good working order. Unfortunately, refined starches such as white flour are largely devoid of such vital nutrients and cannot supply them.

Refined starches are still burned as fuel. But since the food itself is deficient in nutrients, one must draw vitamins and minerals from somewhere else in order to use it. One may call on the body's reserves as long as such reserves exist. But once reserves are depleted, one will begin to withdraw and use up vitamins and minerals from cells that need to retain what they have for their own survival. As a result, those cells will die. The state that exists with respect to the body as a whole at this point is what physiologists call starvation. This process can occur even when one is overweight and consumes many calories—if those calories are "empty calories," unaccompanied by the nutrients needed to metabolize them.

One of the impediments on the part of many people to accepting a diet that is high in starch is the fear that it will cause weight gain. It can, of course, but only if one consumes more starch than one burns. Fat as a fuel can also cause weight gain. But the average person has the impression that starch is worse since there are popular weight loss diets that are based on a high intake of fat and protein, with the total exclusion of starches. Such diets seem more satisfying, because greasy foods stay in the stomach longer. They also can produce a rapid decrease in pounds, but at the same time will often result in a detoxification overload for the kidneys and liver.[65] Interestingly enough, careful investigation of such high-protein, high-fat, meat-based weight-loss diets have shown that though total pounds of body weight decrease, it is primarily water—and in some cases even a small amount of muscle—that is lost. Without realizing it, the dieter maintains fatty tissue while he or she is losing pounds.[66] As soon as the person stops the diet and water returns to the dehydrated tissues, the pounds come back. Most people would probably not consider the whole process to be worth the effort involved if they understood what was going on.

Whole foods—such as whole grains, beans, vegetables, and fruits that are high in complex carbohydrate—are also rich in fiber, and there is some evidence that one may tend to eat fewer calories when on a high-fiber diet.[67] The center in the brain that signals satiation is stimulated by the motions of chewing and swallowing. High-fiber foods, such as whole-grain breads, rice, vegetables, and fruits, tend to require more chewing and swallowing per calorie.

When whole-grain bread and white bread were compared, 10 out of 12 subjects ate less whole-grain bread.[68] When a group of 13 persons were allowed to eat as much as they wished, it was found they ate 22% fewer calories on a diet high in whole grains, vegetables, and other naturally high-fiber foods than when on a diet high in refined carbohydrate. As a result, they lost weight.[69] The residue of high-fiber foods may also pick up and carry out into the stool some of the fats and oils, thereby decreasing their absorption and resulting in a lower caloric uptake.[70, nt.4]

Fat as Fuel

As noted earlier, vegetarian protein coming from grains, legumes, vegetables, and fruits brings along primarily carbohydrate, while animal protein, by contrast, brings along mostly fat. This difference is striking. Even the leanest meat carefully trimmed will contain at the very least 3% fat by weight. This would seem at first like a very small amount, but when one considers the fact that 75% of the meat is water, it can be seen that fat accounts for about 12% of the dry weight. Moreover, since fat is a storage form of energy, it is very dense. While a gram of carbohydrate or

Fat in Lean Meat[25]

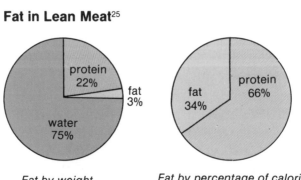

Fat by weight   Fat by percentage of calories

protein accounts for only about 4 calories, for each gram of fat burned 9 calories of energy are produced. Thus in 100 grams of very lean meat, the 3 grams of fat will account for 27 calories, whereas the 20 grams of protein will account for no more than 80 calories. Since there is essentially no carbohydrate in meat, it becomes clear, then, that fat accounts for over a third of the calories in even the leanest cut of meat.

In meat of average fat content, such as regular ground hamburger, the percentage of calories accounted for by the fat will average close to 70%. The amount of fat in so-called "choice cuts" is even higher. Prime beef, for example, is "marbled." This means that there are streaks of fat through the lean part of the meat. This marbling makes the beef tender and more palatable, but it also increases drastically the fat content. If the meat is eaten without trimming it, as is often the case, the fat content is still greater and can easily reach 85% of the calories. (See the table on p. 46.)

Hamburger is notorious for the unreliability of its fat content. Meatcutters often capitalize on their ability to disguise organ meats and trimmings by grinding them into hamburger, and many of these scraps are exceptionally high in fat. Although USDA standards officially limit fat in hamburger to 30% by weight, it has been reported that in practice this may climb to above 60%.[73] A fat content of 65% by weight is roughly the same as 95% of calories. Of course, much of this fat oozes away when burgers are fried, but

Fat in Regular Ground Hamburger [25]

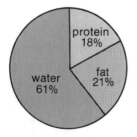

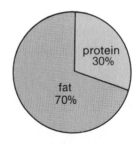

Fat by weight   *Fat by percentage of calories*

ground meat used in meatloaves or casseroles will retain most of it.

Therefore, as a reasonable rule of thumb, one can expect that the average serving of red meat will contain well over half its calories in fat. Unless it is carefully selected and trimmed, this may run to 80% or higher. Even a diet that is otherwise moderately low in fat will become excessively greasy if several servings of such meat are included each day.

One of the few areas in nutrition in which there is a firm consensus is with reference to the advisability of altering fat intake. Although experts on both heart disease[74] and cancer[75-78] agree that the consumption of fats should be cut, doing so is almost impossible as long as fat-rich red meats play a major role in the diet. The goal of fat reduction ranks with the importance of avoiding chemical contaminants and resistant microbes as one of the most compelling health-related reasons to decrease one's intake of meat.

Practical Measures: First Steps in Phase 1

If one has not already done so, a good first step is to limit oneself to a maximum of 2 to 3 red meat meals per week. For many, this represents a significant reduction. It is not uncommon for North Americans to have a meat-based meal 15 or more times a week, since many typical breakfasts, lunches, and dinners are organized around some form of beef or pork. In such a case, reducing pork and beef to 2 or 3 times per week is quite a significant change and really as much as should be attempted in the beginning. Such a step would initiate what we have called Phase 1, which involves the gradual reduction of red meat. Even this should be accomplished slowly. A sudden reduction from 10 to 12 red meat servings a week to 3 or 4 might cause unnecessary discomfort and difficulty.

Since the object is not only to reduce beef and pork but also to reduce the total amount of fats and oils in the diet, one must be careful about what is substituted for the beef and pork that is dropped out. A common catch phrase today is "less red meat, more poultry," and the prospect of fewer meat meals is likely to conjure up a vision of more plates of chicken. However, if we look again at the table on page 46 we will see that poultry, especially if the skin is included, may be as high in fat as some cuts of red meat, or even higher. And if it were fried chicken, then the fat content would climb still higher.

During Phase 1, as the amount of red meat is reduced, poultry and fish may be increased slightly but should not be used at every meal "vacated" by red meat. Rather, it is wise to develop a number of meals that are meatless to replace some of those from which meat has been dropped. Chicken and fish may then move into more prominent places in the diet; that is, they may be used as entrees or as the focus of the more important main meal of the day, rather than appearing in the lighter meals as chicken salad, turkey sandwiches, or fish and chips, for example.

The inclusion of some meatless meals in the course of the day is a very important aspect of the early steps of making a transition to a vegetarian diet. In the beginning, meatless meals should be relatively infrequent and largely restricted to the lighter meals, for example, breakfasts, light lunches, or light suppers. It is reassuring and helpful in the beginning to retain the meat, fish, or fowl entree for the major meal of the day.

But as one proceeds with Phase 1, one may also begin to alter the amount of red meat in the meat meal itself. One way of doing so is to emphasize meat dishes that include other ingredients, so that the meat content can be gradually reduced. Probably the best dishes for this purpose are those that are based in part on legumes, so that part of the protein of the meat can be replaced by that of the legume. An added advantage to such dishes is that they usually involve extensive cooking, so that the danger of infection from microbes carried by the meat is largely eliminated. If a meat/legume dish is selected, one can allow the beans to make up an increasing proportion of the dish, evolving over a period of time into one that is totally vegetarian as well as satisfying and familiar. This is a relatively painless way to make the transition and can involve the progressive exploration of some intriguing ethnic specialties.

A large number of such dishes combine red meats with beans,

such as chili con carne, Brunswick stew, or pork and beans. The principle is simple: the meat with its more familiar appeal is used to flavor the beans, whose taste is less distinct. Most of the recipes for such dishes reflect roughly equal proportions of meat, beans, and vegetables such as onions, garlic, tomatoes, green peppers, or celery, which supply flavor. Seasoning with spices and herbs is a matter of great variation, and often the aspect of the dish that does the most to define its ethnic origin.

Besides stews like chili, meatloaves, burgers, and casseroles, there are other dishes that lend themselves well to combinations of beans and meat. During this phase, small amounts of meat are used, primarily to flavor food. Retaining familiar tastes provides a sense of continuity while allowing plant foods to make up a larger part of the diet. At this stage one is already in good company, having, in effect, adopted the stance of Thomas Jefferson, who wrote: "I have lived temperately, eating little animal food, and not so much as an aliment as a condiment for the vegetables which constitute my principal diet."[79]

When people begin to omit red meat from the diet (or even to decrease the quantity of it) they often express two chief concerns: Without red meat can I get enough protein? and, Can I get enough iron? Though there is widespread anxiety about getting enough protein, and although for the average person protein is almost synonymous with meat, most people feel somewhat reassured by retaining fowl and fish as prominent items in the diet. It's easy to understand that they, too, are rich in protein, and their presence will answer for the time being the concerned friends and relatives who ask, "But where do you get your protein?" If one reduces sweets and other greasy foods as one eliminates meat, and increases more healthful alternatives, such as whole grains and fresh green vegetables, one will gain protein, too. There are also other tricks for increasing protein in the vegetarian diet, such as combining grains and legumes, which will be discussed in the next chapter. However, the question of iron is somewhat more troublesome.

Chili with Meat and/or Beans

½ lb ground beef and/or up to 4 cups cooked beans

1-2 tsp salt

½ tsp pepper

2 T chili powder

1 tsp ground cumin

3 cups peeled, chopped tomatoes

1 medium green pepper, chopped

4 medium onions

Fry onions and ground meat together until onions begin to brown. Add chili powder and green peppers and cook a bit more. Then add other ingredients, bring to a boil, and lower heat. Simmer for about an hour.

The proportion of beans to meat can be varied. As tastes adapt, the beef can be eliminated altogether. As this is done, one may use 2 T olive oil or butter to fry onions, and increase or alter the seasonings somewhat.

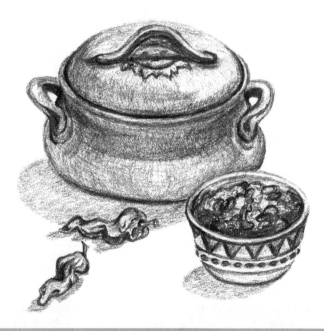

IRON WITHOUT MEAT?

Does the elimination of meat mean one is doomed to become pale and anemic? Is it impossible to be hale, hearty, and red-blooded on a vegetarian diet? There is no question that red meat, such as beef, is richer in iron than many other foods. (See table below.) Yet it is also clear that many plant foods, such as beans and green leafy vegetables, may equal or surpass it. But meat has a special edge in the iron department. Half or more of the iron in muscle meats such as beef is of a sort that nutritionists refer to as "heme" iron. It is found in hemoglobin, the molecule in blood that

Iron Content of Average Portions of Common Foods[nt.5]

Food	Amount	Iron (mg)
Blood sausage	3 oz	17.0
Liver, beef	3 oz	7.5
Beef, sirloin	3 oz	2.5
Fish (Halibut)	3 oz	0.6
Eggs	1 (large)	1.2
Milk (whole)	1 cup	0.1
Kidney beans	½ cup	3.4
Lentils	½ cup	2.1
Navy beans	½ cup	3.8
Whole-wheat bread	1 piece	1.0
Spinach*	¾ cup	2.3
Kale*	¾ cup	1.7
Collards*	¾ cup	0.6
Raisins	2 T	0.6
Molasses	2 T	2.0

*Cooked in own broth until water evaporates (not drained).

Sources: Truesdell et al: *Nutrients in Vegetarian Foods.*[80] U.S. Dept. of Agriculture: *Nutritive Value of American Foods.*[81] Davidson et al: *Human Nutrition and Dietetics.*[82]

turns red on picking up oxygen, and in myoglobin, the pigment that makes muscle tissues red. This iron is assimilated in the body by a different mechanism from that which takes up the iron found in plant foods: the iron-containing fragments of the hemoglobin and myoglobin molecules cross the intestinal wall intact. This seems both to accelerate the absorption of the iron and to protect it from being picked up by, and bound to, substances in the diet that form compounds with iron.[82] For this reason heme iron is absorbed at a rate of from 25% to 35% of what is ingested.[83]

Iron absorption from plant foods, on the other hand, usually runs in the 2% to 10% range.[82,84] Certain iron-binding substances in plant foods, such as the fiber in fruits and vegetables, the phytates of grains, or the oxalic acid in spinach, have been observed to bind iron and are thought to carry it out of the body, preventing the absorption of much of what is present.

The differences in absorption rates between meat and plant foods have led nutritionists to be concerned that vegetarians might be at special risk for iron-deficiency anemia. These fears are not unfounded; in fact, a number of cases of such anemia have been reported among vegetarians.[85-88] That this is a legitimate worry is further underscored by the fact that iron is already one of the nutrients shown by surveys to be low in the diets of many populations, not only in the underdeveloped countries but in the U.S. as well.[89] Those at particular risk are infants, because of the low iron content of milk, children and adolescents, because of their rapid growth, and women during their reproductive years, both because of blood losses during menstruation and because of the demands of pregnancy. For such persons, moving toward a vegetarian diet requires special attention to the issue of iron.

Recently, however, we have learned more about the subtleties of the factors that either inhibit or enhance iron absorption from nonmeat food. Despite earlier opinions to the contrary, recent studies have shown that oxalates[90] and most of the fiber in fruits and vegetables[90,91] when taken in moderate amounts do not interfere with iron absorption in the living body, though some of them may bind iron in the test tube. Phytates, indigestible substances especially concentrated in the bran layer of whole grains, remain controversial.[91-95, nt.6] It's been shown in the case of calcium, as we shall see in the next chapter, that the intestine can develop the ability to break down phytates, thus freeing the mineral bound by them.[96] Whether or not this turns out to be true in the case of iron, other components of bran such as the phosphates it contains do seem to inhibit iron absorption.[97]

However, the effects of one previously suspected inhibitor have definitely been confirmed: that of tea. Black tea is a very potent obstacle to the assimilation of iron. This effect comes from the tannic acid in the tea, which combines with the iron to form an insoluble compound.[90] For this reason, tea probably should not be taken along with meals, though it is possible that some of the traditional additives such as milk or lemon may neutralize the tannic acid and reduce its interference with iron absorption.

Boosting Available Vegetarian Iron

One of the most interesting and important discoveries about iron is that its absorption from grains and legumes can be greatly enhanced by the presence of ascorbic acid (vitamin C). Vitamin C is plentiful in such foods as tomatoes, green peppers, turmeric, and lemons. A recent report states: "The effect of ascorbic acid on non-heme iron absorption has been tested in a number of dietary settings and in every case has been shown to be profound. It plays a particularly critical role in diets in which little or no meat is present."[90] Non-heme iron absorption in one study was quadrupled by including in the meal enough vegetables to provide 65 milligrams of vitamin C.[98] This amount is exceeded by a cup of broccoli or half a green pepper.

Green leafy vegetables, which are often high in both iron and vitamin C, can be exceptionally good sources of dietary iron. Favorite recipes in many parts of the world make generous use of ingredients rich in vitamin C, such as tomatoes, green peppers, or hot chilis. This is especially true of bean dishes (see recipe on p. 140), and it is interesting to discover that legumes such as lentils, beans, and peas have recently been recognized as being particularly rich in iron.[99, 100] The potential of ascorbic acid to facilitate the

Vitamin C Content of Foods Often Used in Vegetarian Meals

Food	Vitamin C mg per ½ cup
Onion	5
Green beans	9
Potato	10
Tomato	25
Spinach	25
Mustard greens	38
Broccoli	50
Kale	75
Green peppers	90
Lemon juice	1T = 7mg

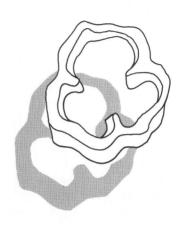

Source: Nutritive Value of American Foods.[81]

assimilation of such iron makes it a valuable source of this mineral for the vegetarian. Lactic acid (in yogurt) has been thought to play a similar role,[101] but other acids probably don't.[98]

There are other tricks for boosting the iron available in nonmeat foods. For example, it has been shown that the iron from pots and skillets can add significantly to absorbable iron in the diet.[102] It is leached from the inside of the pot and combines with the food.[103] Available iron in food can be increased by 100% to 400% when it is prepared in iron cookware.[104] This effect might be excessive when very acidic dishes, such as concentrated tomato sauce, are prepared in iron cookware. The inside of the cooking utensil will lose its shiny surface and the food will become darkened and develop an unpleasant metallic taste. Regular consumption of such food could eventually lead to iron overload. Although a certain amount of iron from cooking utensils is helpful, too much can cause iron to accumulate in tissues and cause illness. Very little iron is carried over into the food when nonacidic dishes are cooked in ironware, especially if some cooking fat is present. Thus, an appropriate rule of thumb for a vegetarian would be to cook about half his food, an assortment of dishes, in iron pots and pans. A heavy iron skillet with beans, peppers, and tomatoes simmering away may be appetizing in part because of the satisfaction of iron needs that it suggests.

Minerals often compete with one another for absorption. Foods very high in calcium can interfere with iron absorption, just as excess iron can interfere with the absorption of other minerals, such as zinc. Too much milk, which is high in calcium and low in iron, can block iron intake.

Researchers Look at Iron in Vegetarians

A number of studies have shown that iron intake among vegetarians is often as high as or higher than that among meat-eaters. [105-110] This is not surprising; if we look again at the iron content of a number of animal and plant foods (see table on p. 64), we see that plant foods are quite rich in iron. Though half the iron in the meat may be heme iron, which is well absorbed, in a well-designed vegetarian diet the vitamin C-rich foods and iron cookware can produce a level of iron intake that is as high or higher, with an availability that is also equal.

Theoretically then, there are good reasons for postulating that a vegetarian could get adequate iron, despite concerns about phytates, oxalates, and fiber. But that's theory. It would be helpful to know what, in fact, is the status of iron in vegetarians as compared with that of the general population.

To find out, researchers studied blood levels of iron and hemoglobin in a group of 56 vegetarian women,[111] since women are at particular risk for iron deficiency, especially during their reproductive years. As might be expected, the iron content of the vegetarians' diets was higher than that in the diets followed by comparable women in the general population. But by accepted methods of estimating the availability of the non-heme iron in plant foods, iron absorption from their diets would be calculated to be quite low, ranging from about 25% to 75% of official recommendations. In view of this, one might expect from such results an iron-deficient and anemic group of women.

Not so. Only 7 of the 56 had hemoglobin concentrations in the blood below 12 milligrams per 100 grams, the point at which one begins to suspect iron deficiency. By comparison, a larger percentage of women in the general population had hemoglobin levels that low. By three separate additional criteria,[nt.7] the vegetarian women were found to have normal levels of iron.

Though some of the vegetarian women took iron supplements or vitamin C, both of which might be expected to boost iron tissue levels, the 25 women who took neither extra iron nor extra vitamin C had hemoglobin and iron levels that were equally as good. This included 9 women who were still menstruating (and therefore regularly losing blood).

The researchers termed the results "surprising." They suggested that the vegetarians had somehow adapted to their diet in such a way as to enable them to increase their efficiency of iron absorption. Although the results may have been due to a skillful combining of food rich in vitamin C with food high in iron, or to the use of iron cookware, it should not astonish us if we also find that long-term vegetarians can handle the iron in plant foods differently from persons accustomed to mixed meat and vegetable diets. Earlier studies done to compare absorption of iron from meat-containing meals with absorption of iron from meals consisting solely of plant foods may not be applicable to those whose digestion has had years to adjust. What's more, if it's true that a well-balanced vegetarian diet is conducive to overall good health, it would not be unlikely that other, as yet unidentified, aspects of metabolism might operate more efficiently, enabling one to use the iron one does absorb in a more effective way.[nt.8]

In any case, it seems clear that one need not become iron deficient on a meat-free diet. But a word of caution: the key qualifier here is "well-balanced." As noted before, simply removing meat guarantees little. The diet must be selected with some care in order to provide for adequate iron nourishment.

There are certain situations in which iron depletion can have serious consequences. One is that of the pregnant woman, where normal development of the fetus depends on adequate iron. Another is that of the child, where too little iron can interfere with mental development during childhood. Infants and preschool children with iron deficiency—even though often showing no signs of anemia—have been found to score lower on intelligence tests and to have a decreased attention span. Replenishing their iron stores with supplementary iron resulted in a prompt improvement in test scores.[114]

But prolonged use of supplements is not the best solution to providing adequate iron. Progressively higher doses of iron given to pregnant women resulted in correspondingly higher levels of hemoglobin and iron in the blood, but also produced progressively lower levels of copper, zinc, and selenium, all of which are also essential minerals.[115] Iron is thought to compete with other minerals for binding sites at the intestinal wall, where absorption takes place. In view of such considerations, it's probably best to supply as much iron as possible through the diet, where it will be present in proper proportions with other essential minerals. Supplements should be reserved for special situations and their use preferably supervised by a professional who can judge accurately how much to give and when to stop.

Summing Up: How to Get Enough Iron

Optimal dietary iron can be provided with a meat-free diet as long as one keeps in mind the following points:
1. The well-planned vegetarian diet (based on whole grains, beans, and green vegetables) has as much iron as the average American diet (or more) but it's less readily absorbed.
2. Absorption can be increased (up to fivefold) by including in the meal fruits and vegetables rich in vitamin C.
3. The iron content of the diet can be doubled, tripled, or quadrupled by using iron pots and skillets.
4. Diets or supplements excessively high in tea (or tannic acid), protein, calcium, phosphorus, or fiber can interfere with iron absorption.

By eliminating meat from the diet and making some associated changes, we can reduce dietary fat markedly, and thus decrease our risk of atherosclerotic cardiovascular diseases and at least some cancers. Moreover, as we shift our caloric intake from fat to carbohydrate, if most of this carbohydrate is derived from whole foods such as grains, beans, fruits, and vegetables, we are also assured a more ample intake of vitamins, minerals, and fiber. It is clear that by using a little ingenuity we can easily attain these very desirable goals without putting our iron status in jeopardy.

SUBSTANTIAL WITHOUT BEING HEAVY

After reading an exhaustive cataloging of the dangers of modern meat, learning of the considerable benefits that accrue upon shifting to a high-fiber, low-fat alternative, and being thoroughly convinced that nutrients such as iron are easily accessible from plant foods, one may still find oneself craving a big juicy steak—at least every now and again. Is the desire for red meat simply an innate and unalterable aspect of humankind's biological nature? Some science writers have maintained that such is the case, pointing out that less than 1% of the world's population voluntarily spurns every type of flesh food.[116] Many of the largely vegetarian people in underdeveloped countries eat little meat because it's simply not available. The affluent classes in such countries generally eat more meat, and meat consumption climbs quickly in countries as they prosper economically.[nt.9] Such a preference for meat might lead to the simple conclusion that man is by nature a carnivore. Humans do not have the extra stomach or rumen of grazers like cows or horses. And we do have canine teeth for tearing meat.

But our canines are quite small compared with those of the true carnivores, such as lions or dogs. Besides, unlike them, we have a mobile jaw, designed for grinding plant foods. We also have an alkaline saliva for digesting carbohydrate, whereas theirs is acidic and best suited to meat. Furthermore, we have a longer intestinal tract than the carnivores, well enough suited to the assimilation of plant foods, though not as long as that of exclusive herbivores.

The truth is, we're omnivores. We're equipped to eat almost any kind of food. This makes us most similar to our closest relatives, the apes and the chimpanzees. They are also omnivores, subsisting quite happily on vegetarian fare for long periods of time. Yet they, too, can be overwhelmed by a hankering after meat: chimps have been observed to eat—besides their usual diet of fruits, leaves, and tree bark—additional nonplant tidbits such as termites, birds' eggs, and, on occasion, the birds, too. In fact, chimps have even been seen killing and eating wild pigs and small baboons.

This is not common, however, and such behavior seems to run in cycles. The flesh-eating lasts a month or two, then seems to wear off. After that, the chimps return to their staple diet of vegetation. Such cycles or crazes of deliberate hunting and meat-eating appear to be stimulated by an accidental or chance capture of prey. This seems to trigger some latent capacity for hunting and killing.[117] It is as though eating the meat activates an instinctual capacity for aggression. There is a time-honored, if not scientifically proven, association between meat-eating and aggressiveness in humans, too. How this might have developed is not difficult to imagine.[118]

Meat and Aggression: A Hypothesis

Though man's early ancestors are thought to have been heavy, rather cumbersome vegetarian food gatherers, changing climatic conditions seem to have reduced the availability of plant foods for long periods, forcing the evolution of a lighter and more stream-lined body capable of running and hunting. The successful stalking and killing of prey must have required the development of cunning and aggression, too. Perhaps this early ancestor of modern man was like his cousin, the chimp, the taste of a kill rekindling his hunting instincts, and gearing him for a period of surviving on animal foods. During other cycles when available food was vegetation, he would appropriately calm down, settling back into a diet of plant foods and a more peaceable way of living.

Such adaptiveness would serve well as long as such a being lived in nature. But agriculture and animal husbandry would create a new set of circumstances. What becomes of the hunter's drive to kill when meat comes from domesticated animals?

Anthropologists have observed that warfare in prehistoric Europe became common only after man began to keep herds of animals for food.[119] It would follow that the consumption of meat by those who live quiet, unaggressive lives could create inclinations to inexplicable violence or a pervasive sense of pointless anger and hostility.

Though such explanations remain largely speculative, they could help account for a number of current psychosocial phenomena that are otherwise baffling, such as sudden outbreaks of violent behavior and the prevalence of anger both overt and suppressed observed by modern psychiatrists working with populations in which meat consumption is high. In any case, it is interesting to note in this connection that for millennia in India meat as an article of diet has been traditionally prescribed for Rajputs, the caste made up of warriors and rulers. By contrast, the Brahmins, who were to dedicate themselves to study and the spiritual life and who were not to engage in battle, were forbidden the use of meat. This lends a bit more support to the hypothesis that man has a dual biological potential and that he can be geared to more aggressive behavior by eating meat. Perhaps over thousands of years of cultural evolution, the people of India discovered how to harness such a potential productively.

Meat and Consciousness

The term *Rajput* is related to *raja,* which means prince or king. It is also related to the word *rajas,* which means the principle of activity or motion. According to traditional ideas that have grown out of the ancient systems of Indian philosophy, certain foods stimulate activity, restlessness, and movement. These are the foods which are *rajasic.* Although red meat in its fresh and most wholesome form is considered to have a predominantly rajasic effect, this is not a principle that can be applied without modification to modern man. In practice, today, as we have discussed, meat is most often not fresh or wholesome and is consumed quite some time and distance from its slaughter. As a result, it is subject to all the problems with spoilage and deterioration that are inherent in a food killed well before consumption. Fruits, grains, vegetables, and beans are different, in that they can be harvested and transported while still alive. They are killed either as they are cooked or as they are eaten. This considerably reduces the opportunity for deterioration.

In the terms of traditional teachings in the Himalayas, food that has undergone some degree of deterioration is considered *tamasic,* and seen as producing a sense of heaviness, lethargy, and irritability in those who eat it. Most fermented foods are included in this category. Fermented meats, such as hams, sausages, and dried beef, would be especially likely to have a tamasic effect. Ready-made foods, whether packaged and frozen or delicatessen-type dishes that have been held under refrigeration for some time, are also likely to have the same drawbacks.

Although the lethargy and heaviness resulting from over-processed, devitalized, and partially deteriorated food is usually felt to be unpleasant, it may, on the other hand, be intentionally induced. After a hectic day (the effects of which are rajasic), the slowing down produced by tamasic foods and beverages may be welcomed. The use of alcohol, which is a fermented tamasic beverage, as a tranquilizing agent is a classic example of this principle put into practice. The use of tamasic foods may produce a similar, though milder and less noticeable, effect.

Becoming accustomed to, or even dependent upon, tamasic foods as a sort of tranquilizer is probably not uncommon. During the transition to vegetarianism, this tendency must be appreciated,

Classification of Foods: Mind/Body Effects

Rajasic	Sattvic	Tamasic
coffee	fresh:	alcohol
tea	milk	meat, aged
spices	fruits	stale food
meat	vegetables	reheated food
fish	grains	overcooked food
eggs	legumes	dried foods
salt	nuts	highly processed
	seeds	foods

since it can sabotage one's best efforts.

But an urge to eat tamasic food may also stem from a lack of good-quality food that is satisfying. One's first attempts to provide oneself with meat-free meals are likely to center around salads, fruits, and lightly cooked vegetables. Although stir fries and rice, as an example, are light and refreshing and are a pleasant change for one who has been used to heavier meat-based meals, one will probably soon tire of them.

Thus, vegetarian meals that are light and unsubstantial, if taken consistently, will lead gradually to an increased craving for heavy animal foods and a tamasic "fix." Therefore one who is involved in the transition to vegetarianism must work systematically during the first phase of this transition to develop the capacity to produce meals that are solid and substantial, without being heavy and dulling.

By the end of Phase 1 it should be possible to completely eliminate red meat from the diet. Phase 1 may take anywhere from a month to a year or more. Poultry and fish will take over as entrees in major meals or in lunches, if that is when one eats out. This usually works out best, since it is often difficult to provide a well-balanced vegetarian meal from the selections available in a restaurant menu. During this phase it is also very important, as emphasized earlier, to learn to plan and prepare a few appealing and substantial meat-free main dishes. Rather than relying heavily on fish, eggs, cheese, fats and oils, or heavily salted condiments to lend appeal, it is better to attain satisfying and substantial meals by cooking foods in a manner that will concentrate them. Vegetables, for example, can be cooked in an open iron skillet, and reduced in bulk. This gives them a "meatier," chewy consistency, so that the density of nutrients is increased, as is the flavor.

It is important to avoid overcooking, as this will result in a tamasic effect and a loss of flavor. Overcooking yields food that is heavy and leaden and that causes one to feel lethargic. Undercooking, on the other hand, will produce food that is bloating, gassy, and prone to produce restlessness and spaciness. Food prepared from fresh, live ingredients, cooked enough but not too much, can be satisfying and substantial, yet leave one both alert and calm. Such food is that traditionally thought of as *sattvic*. The use of food of that quality has been a major goal in many of the great spiritual traditions, since it is recognized as conferring both optimal health and a capacity for expanded consciousness.

Meatless Entrees

As we saw earlier, certain ethnic dishes lend themselves well to the gradual phasing out of their meat content. Such dishes usually involve beans, and since many are of rural or peasant origin, where supplies of meat were seasonal or unreliable, they are flexible. Meat can be included or, if none is at hand, it can be omitted and other ingredients used for seasoning.

By the end of Phase 1, when red meat is totally eliminated, this principle might be expanded. One way of doing so is to devise meatless versions of common meat dishes that may not have any traditional counterpart. Meatless frankfurters and soy-based meat analogues, sold for example as "vegetable cutlets," are now available. Unfortunately, in order to imitate the texture and taste of meat, processes and ingredients are necessary that may detract from the nutritional value of the food.

A less contrived solution is the use of legume-based substitutes that are not intended to be reproductions of meat, but nevertheless replace it to some extent by supplying somewhat similar taste, texture, and appeal.[nt.10] An example would be a lentil loaf, a main dish or entree that could replace meat in a meal that might otherwise remain unaltered. Another example would be a bean ball that is served with spaghetti.

These meatless entrees may not, as we shall see later, be the ultimate in vegetarian eating, but they are often a useful transitional measure. What should be accomplished by the end of Phase 1 is summarized on page 78.

Spaghetti and Bean Balls

1½ cup cooked beans or lentils
(leftover or freshly cooked)

1 cup whole-wheat bread
crumbs

salt to taste

⅛ tsp pepper

1 rounded T grated Romano
cheese

2 eggs lightly beaten

2 T parsley flakes

2 tsp onion powder

Mash beans and mix with other ingredients, adjusting seasonings (less will be needed if leftover, already seasoned beans are used as base). Wet palms, to prevent sticking, and form mixture into walnut-sized balls. Steam on steaming rack 15-20 minutes or bake at 350.° Serve with tomato sauce or with white sauce and mushrooms over spaghetti.

The bean balls can also be seasoned with a little nutmeg and caraway, steamed, and served with an onion or mushroom sauce over rice accompanied by a cooked vegetable, bread, and a salad, as one would serve Swedish meatballs.

For lunches or picnics they can be larger and flatter and can be fried to go into hamburger buns, where they are perfect with lettuce, tomato, and the usual trimmings.

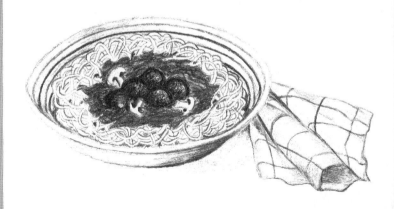

Goals for Phase 1

1. To have eliminated:
- red meat
- refined sugars

2. To have added:
- meatless main dishes at least twice a week (incorporating legume and grain as often as possible)

3. To take regularly:
- a piece of fresh fruit daily
- a green salad at least every other day
- a fresh (not canned or frozen), cooked, green or yellow vegetable at least five days a week
- one serving of a whole grain at least five days a week

PHASE 2

POULTRY

This chapter will focus on the next step in the development of a nutritious, well-balanced vegetarian diet: the elimination of poultry and the systematic increase in vegetable protein. It begins by reviewing the problems that arise when using poultry in the diet, and then moves on to consider the question of how much protein is needed in the diet and how it can best be provided without recourse to meat or poultry. After that we will look at what happens to mineral status with this change; first at calcium metabolism and bone disease on the vegetarian diet, and then at the trace minerals, especially zinc.

The first priority in Phase 2 of the transition to a vegetarian diet is a critical evaluation of the role of poultry in the diet. In America today poultry most often means chicken—fried chicken, baked chicken, broiled chicken, barbecued chicken, and chicken salad, to name some of the more common versions of what has become an increasingly important staple in the American diet. Although other kinds of fowl, such as duck, pheasant, and turkey, also belong in this category, only turkey has even begun to approach the volume of use that characterizes chicken. This is partly because the production of edible chickens has become a streamlined industry. It is now both space- and labor-efficient.

Huge numbers of birds can be produced by modern poultry "factories" where the animals are kept in small spaces, the food is brought in by conveyor belt, and the slaughter, preparation, and packaging are highly automated. Such efficient production techniques have helped make it possible for the price of chicken to be quite low, which probably accounts in part for its continuing growth in popularity.

Whereas the consumption of poultry in 1910 was 18 pounds per person per year,[1] by 1981 it had risen to 63. Currently, although the use of red meat seems to be dropping somewhat, the consumption of poultry continues to climb. Those making changes in their diet for health reasons most often report decreases in beef and pork, while noting an increase in fish and fowl. Though such change may be due in part to economic considerations, there also seems to be a widespread feeling that poultry is lighter and more healthful than red meat. To some extent this may be true: lean, broiled white chicken with the skin removed is certainly lower in fat than lean, broiled trimmed beef.

Classical Ayurveda, the origin and inspiration for much of Oriental and Near Eastern medicine, throws an intriguing light on this question of how different animal foods affect human beings. The peculiar qualities of a specific animal are seen as determining its particular properties as a food: the flesh of the heavy water-dwelling animals like the water buffalo, for example, would tend to increase fluid in the system and produce a feeling of heaviness and lethargy. On the other hand, the consumption of animals from the opposite end of the spectrum, such as birds, especially those from desert habitats, would tend to produce lightness and dryness.

The existence of such subtle effects from animal foods has never been subjected to the scrutiny of modern scientific study. Besides, these effects might be largely irrelevant in the modern world, where methods of raising animals for human consumption so affect the quality of animal foodstuffs that their subtler properties could be obscured. Therefore, despite the fact that its lightness and ease of digestion could provide fowl with inherent advantages over meat, the health of animals raised under the conditions of the modern poultry farm makes them less than desirable as a staple in the diet.

Just as beef cattle and hogs are raised with the use of drugs as growth promoters, so is poultry. Both chickens and turkeys are commonly fed low doses of antibiotics to make them gain more weight. As in the case of the other animals, they also develop resistant strains of microbes.[2] As a matter of fact, salmonella, the bacterium that has been most often associated with foodborne intestinal infections, and the same organism that has produced serious outbreaks of disease in those who have eaten contaminated hamburger, is even more common in poultry than it is in beef.[3] Although plant foods can also harbor and grow salmonella, most infections are carried by animal foods, since animals are the reservoir for the salmonella bacterium. Milk and eggs were formerly a serious problem in this respect, but meat and poultry are now the major identified routes for the transmission of salmonella, and in recent years poultry has surpassed red meat.

Mechanized Poultry Slaughter and Bacterial Contamination

Although both poultry and cattle frequently carry salmonella in their intestinal tracts, the technique used to slaughter and process chickens makes them especially problematic. The birds are shackled by their legs to a conveyor, and then stunned, bled, scalded, defeathered, washed, and eviscerated. Each of these steps contributes to the contamination of the final product, though some cause more spread of microbes than others. As they are shackled and electrically stunned, feces are often shed. During this process, there is considerable contamination back and forth between birds and equipment. The high rates at which the chickens are moved through the production line make it difficult to prevent this. Of 100 cultures taken from a random sampling of equipment surfaces in a typical poultry processing plant, 28 grew salmonella.[4]

The most massive bacterial contamination occurs during defeathering. In earlier times chickens were dressed by hand; after they were dipped in scalding water, the feathers were plucked off manually. Nowadays the whole process is mechanical. Feathers are removed by rubber fingers that flail the bird at a rapid rate. As the machine holds the chicken and the fingers pound it, more bacteria-laden feces are pressed out of the bird, soiling the defeathering machine as well as the chicken and creating a mist or aerosol of airborne microbes that can then spread to adjacent birds and equipment. Over a million microbes per square centimeter can be found on the fingers of the defeathering machine.[nt.1] Chlorine cleaners are only able to reduce this by a factor of 10.[5] These microbes on the skin are beaten by the mechanical flails into the pores vacated by the stripped-off feathers. This increases the number of bacteria in and on the skin by about a hundredfold.[6] Moreover, because of this, the bacteria gain access to channels and crevices below the surface, where they are less affected by heat and tend to resist removal by later washing.[7,8] As knives and machines cut out the entrails of the bird, contamination of the edible parts with organisms such as salmonella further increases.[9] Though washing in a cold bath removes some of the microbes from the surface of the meat, it also serves to cross-contaminate other birds that might not have been infected.[10]

Until recently salmonella was considered the primary disease-causing microbe in meat and poultry. Although it is true that infections with resistant strains of salmonella appear to be on the rise,[11,12] and that poultry is the most common carrier of salmonella, it may harbor another disease-causing organism even more frequently. In some laboratories, this second microbe, a relative newcomer called campylobacter, is the most common pathogen isolated from the stool specimens of patients with acute gastro-intestinal symptoms. Poultry seems particularly prone to contamination with campylobacters;[13] 80% of chickens and 90% of turkeys carried through a typical slaughterhouse produced positive cultures of them.[14] Counts are as high as 100,000 bacteria per bird.[15] Like salmonella, these microbes are present primarily on the surface of the edible parts of the chicken.

The minimum number of bacteria required to produce an acute infection is small. As few as 500 of them have caused illness in susceptible persons.[16] Though cooking kills these organisms, the small numbers needed to cause infection can be transferred from the raw meat to surfaces in the kitchen and then to other foods in the same fashion as that described for beef or pork.

To minimize the risk of transferring campylobacter, as well as salmonella, which is also infective at very low doses,[17] poultry scientists advise using the same precautions for handling raw poultry products that are recommended for red meat. Since proper precautions are not always taken by retailers,[18] meat dishes such as sandwiches or salads that are purchased to be eaten with no further cooking are best avoided. Unfortunately, even nonmeat deli items like rice pudding or macaroni salad are sometimes stored without covering in refrigerators, where drippings from raw meat can contaminate the prepared food.[18]

Thorough cooking is also necessary. Chicken that appears pink and underdone is the most likely source of infection.[19] Since campylobacters survive freezing,[20] inadequate cooking may result from incompletely thawed meat, the inside of which will stay cooler as it is cooked, not reaching high enough temperatures to kill the bacteria.

The symptoms of campylobacter infection are also similar to those that result from salmonella. There is usually abdominal pain, which on occasion may be severe enough to lead the attending physician to suspect acute appendicitis. It would be interesting to know how many emergency operations for presumed appendicitis that turn up normal appendices are actually cases of campylobacter or salmonella infection.

Though both salmonella and campylobacter infections have been reported from very small doses of microbes, it is thought that susceptibility to them will depend on one's state of general health. Whereas as few as 500 bacteria have been shown to cause illness in susceptible persons, such as the aged, the very young, or those who are debilitated or undernourished, healthy young men have ingested up to 200 times that many without developing any symptoms.[21] It would appear that those who follow a diet that is well balanced and rich in nutrients and who have a lifestyle conducive to good health are usually able to ward off all but the more concentrated onslaughts of foodborne bacteria.[22] By contrast, devastating outbreaks of these infections are being reported with alarming frequency in susceptible populations, such as the residents of nursing homes.

A Cancer-Related Microbe in Poultry?

The potential for drug-resistant intestinal infections from poultry is beginning to be more widely recognized by public health officials and food scientists. But there is an even darker side to the poultry question—one that has been raised by a small number of researchers who have consistently identified and grown out a microbe from chickens that produces malignant growths in other experimental animals. It has to do with a possible link between unhealthy chickens and cancer in humans.

This organism, different from bacteria like salmonella or campylobacter, has been recultured from the tumors produced, and identified again as the same microbe. This stepwise process satisfies all the criteria required by scientists for establishing the causal role of a microorganism in a disease. The organism is described as atypical, in some ways like a virus, in others like a bacterium, and is not easily studied using standard laboratory techniques. For this reason, it is felt, the organism has escaped the notice of most cancer researchers.

Actually the microbe described by this group of scientists is thought to be identical to that originally demonstrated in poultry cancers by Dr. Peyton Rous in 1910. In the following decades Dr. Rous refined and confirmed his findings on the transmissable nature of this cancer-related microbe and in 1966 he was awarded the Nobel Prize for this work. Though the extent to which such infections are involved in human cancer remains controversial, Dr. Rous and others have remained concerned that the risk of cancer being transmitted by infected poultry is serious and widespread.[23-25]

Phasing Out Poultry

In any case, the risk of contamination with antibiotic-resistant bacteria is in itself sufficient cause for adding poultry to beef and pork on the list of dietary undesirables. A recent study documented multiple drug resistances in 80% of 3,500 cultures of salmonella taken from such food-producing animals.[26]

Moreover, dropping poultry provides some other important

advantages, too. By eliminating fowl in addition to red meat, we are able to further decrease the total intake of flesh food in the diet. This permits us to bring down fat consumption another notch or two, since most chicken dishes contain quite a sizeable percentage of fat calories (see table on p. 46). It also allows us to decrease animal protein and our intake of chemical toxins, as well as possible undesirable microbes. Moreover, we can then, by replacing these animal foods with plant foods, increase vegetable protein, complex carbohydrate, fiber, and vitamins and minerals—all desirable goals.

As with red meat, the first steps toward eliminating poultry can be taken by preparing dishes that contain less amounts of the animal food. Once more, this is most ideally accomplished by adding beans. The beans allow one to begin to move away from animal protein by basing the diet on a foundation of grains and legumes. Unlike red meat, poultry combines best with the more mildly flavored beans. White beans and pea beans go better with the delicate white meat, while lentils blend well with the darker parts. Bean/poultry dishes are well suited to serving over rice, or when made with a cream sauce, over toast.

As one moves away from the use of poultry, anxiety about the ability to obtain enough protein often arises. To deal with such concerns, we will first consider the principles of combining plant proteins skillfully so as to maximize their value, and then discuss the question of how much total protein is needed each day.

AMINO ACIDS: COMPLEMENTATION VERSUS SUPPLEMENTATION

Although meat, fish, and dairy products are thought of as protein foods—and we may on occasion acknowledge that beans or nuts have protein—we often fail to notice that other plant foods have protein too, such as grains or green leafy vegetables. Even fruits have some protein; a few, like oranges, contain rather generous amounts. But plant foods are different from animal foods as far as their protein is concerned. First of all, there's less of it. While a fourth to a half of the calories in beef may be from

White Beans and Chicken

1/2 lb (1 cup) white beans
  (e.g., Great Northern)
  (3 cups cooked)

2-4 T butter or olive oil

1/2 tsp poultry seasoning (or
  sage or thyme)

1 clove garlic, minced

salt and pepper to taste

3 large chicken breasts,
  skinned, boiled, and boned

Soak beans overnight, then drain. Skim fat from chicken broth, discard, and add broth to beans. Cook, adding boiling broth or water as necessary, but allow most liquid to cook away. Sauté chicken briefly in butter or oil. Add garlic and herbs and saute another few minutes. Then add beans, salt, and pepper, cover and cook on low heat for 5-10 minutes to allow flavors to mix. Serve with rice, a cooked green vegetable, and bread.

As the amount of chicken is reduced, the amounts of beans and butter or oil are increased, until a full pound of beans and 4 T of butter or oil are used. Tofu can be substituted for part or all of the chicken.

With or without the chicken, this dish can be dressed up by sautéing 2 cups of sliced mushrooms before the garlic and herbs are added, and by pouring in 1/2 to 2/3 cup white wine along with the beans.

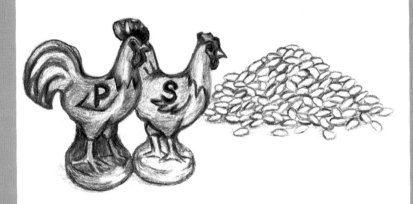

protein, only a little more than a tenth of those in wheat are. Even soybeans, the most protein-rich of the legumes, are only one-quarter protein. This alone is not a serious problem, since most of the rest of plant foods is carbohydrate, which is, as we saw, a very desirable fuel. But there's another major difference between the protein of plant and animal foods, and that has to do with its quality.

To understand the issue of protein quality we must first look at how proteins are made. A protein molecule is essentially a chain. The links in this chain are the smaller molecules called amino acids, each of which contains a nitrogen atom.

The amino acid unit itself has two characteristic parts, the first of which makes it an acid and the second of which contains nitrogen and is indicated by the term *amino.* This word comes from the same root as *ammonia,* the nitrogenous gas given off by decaying protein or by the perspiration of someone who eats a high-protein diet. The nitrogen, which makes protein unique among the large molecules found in biological systems, comes ultimately from the atmosphere. Air is approximately 80% nitrogen, the rest being primarily carbon dioxide and oxygen. Although most plants must take their nitrogen from other decaying plant or animal material in the soil, a few—primarily the legumes—are able to "fix" nitrogen taken from the air. Special bacteria around their roots make this process possible, and the seeds of these plants are particularly rich in the nitrogen-containing protein.

Essential Amino Acids

A total of 22 amino acids can be found in the body, and most of these can be broken down and reassembled into others. There are, however, 8 that the body is unable to manufacture. These 8 amino acids must be taken into the body preformed, and for this reason they are called "essential." (There may be a few others that are necessary in small amounts, especially for newborn infants.) Like vitamins and minerals, they must be present in the diet or one will show signs of deficiency. Moreover, to be best utilized, these 8 must be available in the proper proportions, that is, the proportions in which they are used to produce the common protein molecules of the body. One of the most important of such proteins is albumin, which is manufactured in the liver cells and circulated in the blood. It is in this form that protein is picked up by other cells to be used as needed. Thus egg white, which is a form of albumin, was found by researchers to be one of the best utilized of common proteins and was often taken as a standard for the ideal proportions of essential amino acids (EAAs). More recent and detailed experiments have refined our ideas about what constitutes an optimal balance of amino acids. A standard that is currently in wide use is that shown in the table below.[nt.2]

If one of the essential amino acids is present in a food in very small quantities, then the body's ability to use the protein in that food is limited by the shortage of that particular amino acid. Because of the lack of it the cells are hindered in their ability to assemble the other remaining amino acids from that food into the chains or protein molecules that are needed to sustain life. The amino acid in that supply then becomes the "limiting amino acid." The basic issue with protein, therefore, is not merely how much a

Ideal Essential Amino Acid Pattern
(mg per gram of protein)

Isoleucine	40
Leucine	70
Lysine	55
Methionine (and Cystine)*	35
Phenylalanine (and Tyrosine)*	60
Threonine	40
Tryptophan	10
Valine	50

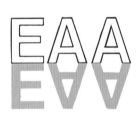

*Cystine can be used to help satisfy some of the need for methionine, so the amount of cystine present is added to that of methionine. A similar principle applies to phenylalanine and tyrosine.[nt.3]

Source: Hackler: *In Vitro Indices,*[27] p. 57.

person gets, but whether what he gets contains the 8 essential amino acids in the proper proportions, or whether its use is seriously limited by a shortage of one or more of them.

A balanced combination of amino acids, such as that found in egg white, can be well utilized with no wastage. The amino acid pattern of meat protein is very similar to that of egg white. The same is true of fish, poultry, or milk (see table below). But most plant foods, when looked at individually, are relatively deficient in one or more of the essential amino acids, and therefore the utilization of their protein is not as efficient. A certain percentage of it won't be used as protein; instead, it is burned as fuel or gotten rid of. For this reason it is said to be of poor quality.

Corn, for example, varies from 6% to 12% protein[29, 30] but, of this, only about half is usable since corn protein is quite low in a couple of the essential amino acids (lysine and tryptophan).

Essential Amino Acid Content of Common Proteins Shown as Percentage of Ideal

	Ideal	Egg white	Chicken	Fish	Milk	Soy	Rice	Lentils	Wheat bread	Spinach	Beans (mung)	Collards	Corn	Peanuts
Isoleucine	100	156	133	127	145	147	117	133	126	115	137	78	115	117
Leucine	100	124	103	108	153	121	124	100	112	110	128	80	186	99
Lysine	100	109	160	160	153	126	80	111	48	112	124	94	53	74
Methionine + Cystine	100	180	114	122	103	98	91	44	115	106	49	77	91	77
Phenylalanine + Tyrosine	100	175	125	106	180	148	161	118	138	125	107	117	178	165
Threonine	100	110	108	107	118	107	98	90	83	110	76	73	100	77
Tryptophan	100	150	120	100	180	151	110	90	107	160	70	141	60	126
Valine	100	158	98	106	116	115	142	108	102	110	118	100	102	139
		98				98	80	44	48		49	73	53	74

% of ideal of limiting EAA (= chemical score)

Sources: Hackler: *In Vitro Indices,*[27] pp. 46-65. Orr & Watt, *Amino Acid Content of Foods,*[28] p. 57.

Proportion of Protein That Can Be Used as Protein in Various Plant Foods

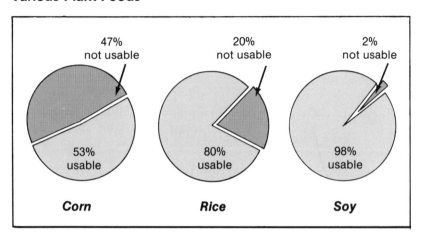

Therefore we must consider that only 3% to 6% of the energy from corn is protein that can serve the body's needs. Though we will discuss later in some detail the exact amount of protein one should take in each day, a rough estimate is that 6% of the energy intake should be high-quality protein. Only that corn which has the highest protein content (12%) would make the grade, and then only barely.

Because of their amino acid makeup and the relatively poor utilization of their protein, most grains are unreliable as the sole source of protein. This would seem a serious problem when one remembers that grains are the staple on which most vegetarian diets are based. Indeed, it was primarily because of such reasoning that nutritionists long considered vegetarian diets incapable of supporting good health. This conclusion would be justified if vegetarians relied on only one plant food, such as a grain, for their entire dietary intake.[nt.4] If half the protein of such a diet were unusable because of a lack of one of the essential amino acids, then one might well become protein deficient.

Combining Plant Foods for Protein Excellence

But, of course, no one eats only a single food, at least not by choice. We eat combinations of foods, and fortunately not all

Complementary Amino Acids

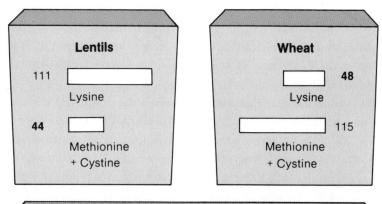

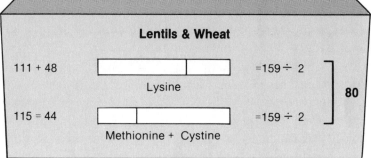

Chemical scores for lentils and wheat alone are, respectively,
44 and 48. Together they are 80—nearly twice as much protein can
be used when they are combined.

plant foods are low in the same amino acids. While one plant food
may be deficient in one amino acid, a second food will most likely
be low in a different one. Moreover, most foods not only have
relative deficiencies of one or more essential amino acids, they
usually have relative excesses of others. For example in the table
on page 89, we see that wheat is somewhat low in threonine, and
quite low in lysine, but has methionine and cysteine to spare. When
we eat a variety of plant foods, the surplus of essential amino acids
in one vegetable or grain tends to make up for the deficiency of
those amino acids in the accompanying food.

Such is the case with lentils, which have quite different
patterns of deficiency and surplus. They contrast with wheat

in a way that is typical of grains and beans. Wheat, like most other grains, is relatively poor in lysine.[nt.5] Lentils, on the other hand, come out quite well in the lysine department but make a bad showing, as do most legumes, when it comes to methionine. But the amino acid patterns of these two—wheat and lentils—mesh nicely.

Experiments with laboratory animals have shown what a dramatic difference combining plant foods can make. Feeding a diet of 18% protein, an ample amount by most standards, failed to produce good growth when the protein was derived from wheat only. The same thing happened when the wheat was left out but enough lentils added to bring the protein level up to the same 18%. In neither case was growth up to usual standards. But animals on a third diet, using a combination of both proteins, did surprisingly

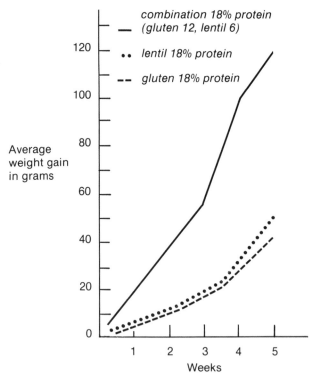

Differences in Growth Rate with Different Protein Sources

Source: Life and Health.[32]

better. The total amount of protein was still the same 18% of caloric intake, but this time it was part wheat protein and part lentil protein. With the protein derived from a combination of wheat and lentils, the animals' growth was almost tripled.[32] When nearly three times as much benefit can be gained from the identical quantity of protein by changing its source, and therefore its quality, in this fashion, combining plant foods knowledgeably is clearly of great value.

This special synergistic effect is found most commonly as a result of the combining of a grain and a legume.[nt.6] It is generally termed "complementarity." Though even eating a randomly varied vegetarian diet will boost the quality of the protein available to some extent, this benefit can be magnified if one understands which foods to combine with each other, and does so skillfully.

Although the most frequently used and, in many ways, the most valuable combination is that of grain and legume, certain other combinations are also quite helpful too, such as grains and milk. The low lysine content of wheat can be helped by milk, which

True Complementation
based on responses to varying the ratio of two proteins without changing the total protein intake

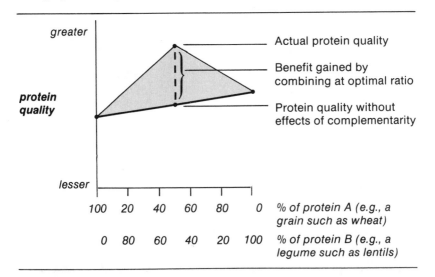

Source: Bressani: *Protein Supplementation.*[33]

contains a generous portion of extra lysine. This improves the value of the wheat protein. Moreover, the wheat has a relative surplus of methionine, the least abundant essential amino acid in milk.[nt.7] (See table on p. 89.) Therefore the combination is complementary; but this combination will never have a better-quality protein than that of milk itself. This is in contrast to the grain/legume combination, where the quality of the combined protein is far superior to the quality of an equal amount of either grain or legume protein alone. The synergistic meshing of deficiencies and surpluses seen with grain/legume combinations is termed true complementation by nutritionists. (See illustration on p. 93.) The less dramatic effects resulting from a combination like wheat and milk, in which the quality of the better of the proteins serves as a ceiling or upper limit, has been called partial complementation. (See illustration below.) In both these types of complementary pairs, the proportions of each of the two protein foods being combined is important.

Partial Complementation
based on responses to varying the ratio of two proteins without changing the total protein intake

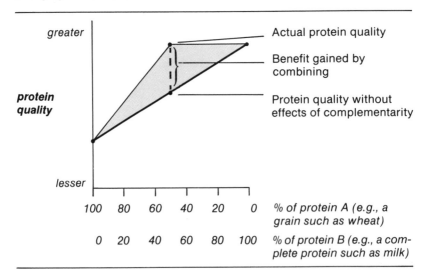

Source: Bressani: *Protein Supplementation.*[33]

The protein that cannot be used to make protein chains in the body because of the lack of certain essential amino acid links is converted to a form that can be burned as fuel. This involves removing the amine or nitrogen portion of the amino acid, a process called "deamination." The cast-off amine fragments are wastes and must be excreted through the efforts of the kidneys and the liver. A healthy, robust person can handle a good deal of such a "deamination burden," but if kidney or liver function is impaired the wastes can overwhelm and irritate the organ, accumulate in the body, and impair physical and mental activity. For this reason it is customary to put patients with renal or liver disease on carefully regulated low-protein diets. Unfortunately, due to sedentary lifestyles and the frequent use of alcohol, caffeine, and diets rich in fats, oil, and sugar, it is the author's clinical impression that many persons today are suffering from mild and undiagnosed, but nevertheless significant, disability of the liver or the kidneys, or both the liver and the kidneys. A lot of poor-quality protein is not a happy choice in such a situation, as such protein must be deaminated, further burdening the disabled organs.

Although most frequently used combinations of plant foods, especially those evolved over long periods of time in stable ethnic traditions, have arrived at good balances of essential amino acids, some of our more modern innovations are less successful. The peanut butter sandwich, for example, a relatively recent American invention, teams up two proteins, those of wheat and peanuts, that are seriously deficient in the same essential amino acids: lysine and threonine (see table on p. 89). The percentage of the protein contained here that can be used is only about 68%, so the deamination burden is rather heavy.

For such reasons it is useful to know how to combine proteins effectively. With beans and rice, for example, there is an optimal ratio. If more beans are added beyond that ideal proportion, protein quality drops off again, as is suggested by the diagram on page 93, and the deamination burden increases. Though in general the quantity of grain should be substantially more than the quantity of beans, the ratios can vary over a considerable range.[33] Black beans need be served only in small quantities with white rice, and indeed that is the custom in Latin America, where this combination is an ethnic favorite. On the other hand, in the southern states of the U.S., cornbread and black-eyed peas will appear on the table in nearly equal quantities, and according to researchers, that is the ratio that is optimal. Wheat flour and milk protein also reach their maximal complementarity in roughly equal proportions, and that's probably right on target for a cheese sandwich or a bowl of cream of wheat cooked in milk.

The Role of Soy—and of "Ordinary Beans"

Despite the fact that soybeans are a legume, the combination of soy with many grains,[nt.8] such as rice and corn, is regarded as only partial complementation. This is because soybeans are atypical. Their amino acid content is closer to ideal than that of most beans and peas (see table on p. 89); that is, they are less deficient in their limiting essential amino acids (methionine and cystine) than are other legumes. This means that soy protein can stand alone as a source of protein in the diet better than can the proteins of other legumes, such as lentils, mung beans, or garbanzos. Although soy may sometimes be used to improve the protein quality of a grain, it does not itself benefit significantly from the combination, since it's not seriously deficient. For this reason, soy products might be thought of as similar to milk. Both of them can function in the same way we saw milk helping wheat, to provide partial complementation, boosting the quality of protein in the grain, but benefiting little themselves.

Or they can function in a different way by simply adding extra protein. That is what happens when a milk product such as cheese is added to a meal that already has a good balance of amino acids. In this case the protein is simply a supplemental additive; rather than its amino acid pattern complementing that of what it's added to, it merely exists alongside it in the meal, supplying its own, additional protein. Such a supplement can be added on top of a combination of a grain and an ordinary legume, since the combination is already a reasonably good protein. In such a case, there is no optimal ratio between one protein source and the other, as there is with complementation; thus, one need not be preoccupied with proportions in cooking and serving. Hence, a little cheese or tofu, for example, can be added to any meal whenever it is convenient, available, and needed to bolster overall protein intake. Soy products such as tofu are, therefore, excellent "protein boosters," and are preferably used that way rather than being used to replace other legumes that should be regularly served along with grains as a sort of inviolable marriage.

There are additional reasons, too, that soybeans should not be allowed to displace other legumes, despite the convenience and the availability of the burgeoning variety of "soy foods." Soybeans (and most soy products) are relatively high in fat (see table on p. 105.) For that reason, tofu is not among the best antiatherosclerotic items in the diet. Other legumes apparently are, however. In fact, ordinary legumes lead the list of foods that are currently being discovered to have potent effects in the prevention of diseases such as heart attacks,[34-36] cancer,[37] and diabetes, and in the treatment of hypoglycemia.[38]

The metabolism of legumes results in less abrupt increases in sugar, which means less of a need for sudden outputs of insulin and consequently less strain on the insulin-secreting cells of the pancreas.

The combination of grains and beans may be even more effective than the beans alone in preventing some of these diseases. In one research study, more beans and rice were correlated with cleaner coronary arteries—regardless of the amount of meat in the diet.[39] In any event, combinations such as rice and beans seem an appropriate foundation for a vegetarian menu. As many ethnic traditions demonstrate, they are often the protein backbone of the low-meat or meat-free diet; they not only replace animal foods that carry health risks, but bring benefits all their own. In fact, the addition of grain/legume combinations to the diet may turn out to be a health imperative, whether one is aiming to become vegetarian or not.

Beyond Grain/Legume Combinations

Even so, a simple grain/legume formula is not the total answer to the vegetarian's protein needs. A steaming dish of rice and lentils may be time-honored and even mouth-watering, but it remains low in certain essential amino acids, especially methionine (see table on p. 89). Adding wheat bread to this meal does much for its methionine content, but threonine still lags.

The truth is, of course, that beans and rice, even when accompanied by bread, are seldom considered a full or balanced vegetarian meal, as anyone who is familiar with ethnic dishes will attest. Green vegetables are a coveted adjunct, and are always included when they can be found. Not only do the vegetables provide the vitamin C that enhances iron absorption, as detailed in the preceding chapter, but also on occasion they may do wonders for the essential amino acid balance of the meal's protein. Spinach, for example, helps supply the threonine missing from the meal of lentils, rice, and bread, as would a bit of milk or cheese cooked into the dish.[nt.9]

Stringing together so many protein elements in a meal in a coordinated and well-orchestrated manner may seem a bit overwhelming, and protein is only one of the nutrients that must be attended to. Though theoretically the combining of complementary amino acids is straightforward, when studies are done for protein utilization the results only roughly approximate what one would expect from the theory.[40]

One might conclude, then, that although it is true that modern research has clearly validated the common practice of putting together plant proteins such as grains and legumes, there's still more to be learned about protein combinations. Approaching the cafeteria line with a pocket calculator and an amino acid table is not conducive to good digestion anyway. What should be gained from this discussion is not a mechanical application of amino acid ratios but a respect for traditional diets and a heightened interest in other dietary patterns that have been commonly followed and that are frequently correlated with good health.

A study done recently in India showed vegetarian children to be taller and heavier than their meat-eating counterparts.[41] Nutritionists were surprised, since studies in the U.S. and Britain had found vegetarian children to be underweight and below norms for height.[42,43] They suggested that the more robust appearance of the vegetarian children in India[nt.10] might be due to differences in hygiene, since it is difficult in a warm climate to prevent meat from spoiling and transmitting diseases, and it was noted that the vegetarian children were sick less often than those who ate meat. But another and perhaps equally valid explanation is that the Indian mother understands better such crucial principles of vegetarian nutrition as combining grains, legumes, and vegetables. Such combinations are the basis of the Indian vegetarian diet.

Although vegetarians in the West are coming gradually to appreciate this point more, they still tend to emphasize vegetarian versions of meat meals, such as spaghetti (without the meatballs—or bean balls, for that matter), ratatouille, or rice and stir-fried vegetables. In imitating the meat menu without the meat, one runs the risk of omitting important elements that belong in the meal. The most obvious and frequent example is the omission of legumes.

Beans are overlooked in part because their proper preparation is rarely understood. This is a formidable challenge, since considerable skill is needed to produce a bean dish that is both delicious and digestible. It's certainly possible, as many ethnic specialties from around the world amply demonstrate, but too often, attempts by the untrained produce bean dishes that are bland, chalky, and gassy.

A vegetarian diet based on grain/legume combinations, low in fat and sugar, and rich in green vegetables (especially cooked leafy ones), is off to a good start. The protein content of such a diet can be supplemented as much as necessary through the addition of tofu, milk products, or, if one wishes, eggs or seafood. Nevertheless, although supplementation may be critical, it can also be overdone. Protein intake should be knowledgeably regulated. In order to be able to do so, it will be helpful to explore more fully the question of protein requirements. The answers are somewhat complex. The precise amount of protein needed by any given

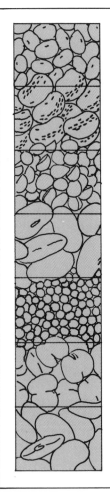

How to Make Beans Less Gassy

1. Generally, smaller beans are more digestible (e.g., mung beans as compared with kidney beans).
2. Soak overnight, then discard soaking water. This eliminates some gas-forming substances and brings beans out of dormancy.
3. Cook until well done—beans should be soft enough to mash between fingers.
4. If water is added during cooking, it should be boiling hot.
5. Season with spices like turmeric, cumin, coriander, ginger, black mustard seeds, cardamom, cloves, and black pepper, and herbs such a bay leaves, thyme, sage, and marjoram. Onions or garlic, or both, also help stimulate digestion.
6. Add salt and fat or oil unless contraindicated.
7. Near end of cooking add acid seasonings such as tomato or lemon juice and allow to simmer 10 to 15 minutes more.
8. Cook with enough water to make a dilute dish and serve in small quantities with the appropriate proportion of grains such as rice.

person is not so easily determined. There are a number of factors that must be considered, and experts are not unanimous on how to allow for them all.

HOW MUCH PROTEIN?

The proteins of the body are of two types: fibrous and globular. The fibrous protein molecules provide the structural framework for the tissues, constituting the basis of connective tissue, of skin, and of the network within which minerals are deposited to make bone. Strands of some of these proteins are bundled together to form muscle fibers, while others make up tendons, ligaments, and even hair and nails. The globular proteins circulate in the blood and tissue fluids either as globulins, which are antibodies, or as albumins and enzymes. Some of these proteins are broken down and rebuilt more frequently than others. For example, it is thought that the lining of the small intestine is renewed every 24 to 48 hours, whereas connective tissues such as ligaments and fascia are much more stable.

Though an adult man may manufacture upwards of 200 grams of protein a day, most of this, probably 80%, is recycled—it is made by reassembling the amino acids that come from the breakdown of body proteins that are being replaced. The other 20% is lost and must be supplied afresh, from the diet. If it is not forthcoming, the body begins to go into negative nitrogen balance: more nitrogen is lost through the excretion of wastes than is taken in through diet. When this happens, sound protein structures must be broken down and sacrificed to provide the protein needed to continue vital life processes. A person in this state is said to be protein deficient.

Protein deficiency is real enough and can occur in vegetarians who don't understand the principles of providing protein from a diet without meat. How far afield one can stray is illustrated by the contemporary teenager who, having abruptly "gone vegetarian," arrives at his favorite hangout and orders french fries and a soda but no burger.

While this example may represent a sort of caricature of the modern vegetarian, less extreme versions of the same error no doubt abound. Where meat is a reliable and rich source of protein, it is not uncommon for the other items in the meal to be low in protein. Dropping the meat out of such a meal leaves a huge void in the protein department. A meat-eater without meat does not a vegetarian make—at least not a healthy one.

The Protein Habit

Yet it is also true that protein can be overdone. A heavy intake of animal protein produces a sort of energizing or stimulating effect of the type that we have termed rajasic in the preceding chapter. Physiologists talk about the "specific dynamic action" of protein: that is, when protein is metabolized, a certain percentage of its caloric value is consumed by its own processing and seems to produce some heat. Thus body-builders who consume very high-protein diets in an attempt to increase muscle bulk may have an intolerance for warm rooms, sweat profusely, and be loaded with nervous energy. Carbohydrate doesn't have this effect.

Irritant or stimulant effects from meat might also come from substances that accumulate in meat tissues after slaughter. Or perhaps they are simply due to the relatively high intake of protein that is common on a typical meat diet. Whatever the cause, when one stops meat, especially if one's consumption of it has been considerable, he or she may feel a letdown similar to that which follows when someone who is accustomed to drinking coffee stops suddenly. (This does not, of course, mean that the human body requires coffee; it simply means that one has become habituated to its effects and dependent on them.)

For the person who is interested in improving his diet and health it is important to be aware of this phenomenon, so that if he encounters such an effect along about the middle of Phase 2 he will understand why it is happening and understand how he can remedy it. Otherwise it may lead to a progressive craving for protein, or sugar, or caffeine, or anything else that might replace the stimulation that has been lost. This protein withdrawal may, in fact, be one of the major obstacles to the gradual elimination of animal foods from the diet. When one encounters this sense of letdown one may be tempted to conclude, "I'm a person who needs meat in my diet. That's just the way my metabolism works."

One may also find oneself missing the sense of fullness that follows a high-protein and high-fat meat meal. Since fat and protein both delay gastric emptying time, a substantial serving of meat will ensure that the stomach remains occupied for many hours. Vegetable foods, unless fortified with extra fat and added protein, will move on more quickly. That is why the typical meat-eater will complain, "I like Chinese food, but an hour later I'm hungry again!" The emptying of the stomach is misinterpreted as hunger. Westernized Chinese restaurants have discovered they can squelch such complaints and hang on to their meat-eating clientele by using more meat and less vegetables and by drenching their food with fats and oils.

Meat withdrawal symptoms can be countered by making the transition away from meat and poultry more gradual and by ensuring an adequate intake of vegetable protein. It's important to allow the body time to regear itself so that one can begin to get a sense of what it's like to function on the basis of a natural, spontaneous, and even energy, without depending on a diet high in animal protein to provide a combination of fullness and stimulation.

Learning to enjoy the lightness of a digestive tract that is at rest, and the energy that derives from the food, and learning not to feel alarmed that one's stomach is empty or that one has no stimulant on board is an extremely important aspect of the transitional process. Failure to make this shift in attitude may doom the whole effort to become vegetarian, or it may result in succumbing to one of the three great pitfalls that await the aspiring vegetarian: the cheese temptation, the granola habit, and the peanut/nut obsession.

Cheese and Granola

In casting about for something to take the place of animal foods, cheese is a prime candidate, since it is also a source of concentrated protein and fat. A slab of cheese may be as filling and stimulating as a piece of steak, but it is also as rich in fat—in some cases richer—and as a result it is heavy and slow to digest. Cheese also tends to be constipating. For both these reasons it should never be taken in large quantities. Moreover, since aged cheeses are fermented, they run the risk of being contaminated with undesirable organisms or their by-products, and are liable to create the irritating, lethargic, tamasic effects referred to earlier in regard to meat.

Granola is another frequent target for the cravings of one who is withdrawing from meat. Though it is made from whole grains, it is often high in sugar and vegetable oils, which keep fat levels up and also carry other risks as well, as we shall see later. In making granola, the grain is coated with vegetable oil and then roasted—a process that often raises the oil to a temperature at which its molecules combine with one another to form polymers. Polymerized vegetable oil is what constitutes the durable film produced by paint or varnish as it dries. Such a film on the grains of granola is difficult for digestive juices to penetrate. Thus it's not surprising that granola will remain in the stomach a long time, replacing the sense of fullness and heaviness that is lost when meat is eliminated. Though it may be considered useful in this role, at least as a temporary expedient, most people eventually find it too heavy and burdensome to deserve a prominent place in a healthful vegetarian diet.

Peanuts and Nuts

Another much-abused meat substitute is peanut butter. A person who has cut down on his meat intake will often confess to craving peanuts and peanut butter. As we've seen, the protein in peanuts is not of very good quality, even when combined with bread. What's more, peanuts are also quite high in oil, as are other nuts. Many nuts, such as walnuts and pecans, will, like some meats and cheeses, contain close to 90% fats, and for this reason are not a good source for one's major protein intake. Other nuts, such as cashews and almonds, as well as seeds like sunflower and sesame seeds, though somewhat less oily, will still have 70% to 80% of their calories as fats.

The high fat and oil content of nuts, combined with their hard texture, make them difficult to chew up into particles small enough to digest easily, and eating more than a small amount of nuts can be very burdensome to the liver and kidneys. In the Ayurvedic tradition, one is cautioned against taking more than a couple of

Fat Content of Beans, Nuts, and Other Foods: Percentage of Calories as Fats and Oils

	Beans & Peas	Dairy Products	Meat & Poultry	Nuts & Seeds
Above 80%		Cream cheese 91%	Pork sausage 86%	Pecans 97% Walnuts 91% Almonds 85% Peanut butter 81%
60-80%		Most cheeses 60-75%	Hamburger* 75%	Cashews 77% Sunflower seeds 76%
40-60%	Tofu 55% Soybeans 41%	Whole milk 51%	Chicken 40-50%	
20-40%		Lowfat (2%) milk 32%		
Below 20%	Garbanzos 12% Most beans† 2-4% Lima, kidney 4% Lentils, mung 3%	Skim milk 0%		

*See discussion on pp. 58-60.
†See nt. 3, p. 259.

Source: U.S. Dept. of Agriculture: *Nutritive Value of American Foods.*[44]

nuts at a time, and in traditional diets nuts are used in small quantities, usually cooked into grain and legume dishes or used sparingly as a garnish. They can also be ground into a paste and mixed with milk curd to form a spread that contains an excellent balance of amino acids[45] and combines with whole-grain bread to provide a very satisfying source of protein for one who is vegetarian. (See recipe below.)

Compared to most nuts, peanuts are relatively perishable. They have a strong propensity for growing a problematic strain of mold called aspergillus flavus, which in turn produces a substance called aflatoxin.[46] Aflatoxin is one of the most toxic agents found in nature. Animal studies have shown that short-term exposure to substantial levels of aflatoxins can result in acute toxicity; chronic low-level exposure can cause liver cancer.[47] Once moldy peanuts are roasted, however, it is not apparent that they have been contaminated, and they may be used for food anyhow. A small percentage of peanut butters of all sorts are periodically found to be contaminated with aflatoxins.[nt. 11]

Paneer Spread

Roast equal amounts of cashews, blanched almonds, and sunflower seeds until light golden brown. Put in a blender and grind till a coarse meal, then add an equal volume of fresh low-fat paneer (cottage cheese made with lemon), and enough boiled milk to be able to blend into a thick nut-butter consistency. It may be made either smooth or crunchy. Refrigerated, it will keep several days.

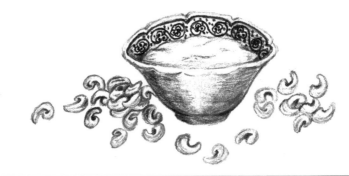

Peanuts, of course, are not botanically nuts. It is the term *pea* in the name that should receive the emphasis, since peanuts are legumes. They differ from other legumes like lentils, kidney beans, and chick peas, however, by growing underground. They also differ by being higher in fat and, as we have seen, by having a type of protein that is inadequate in the same way as that of grains, so that grains and peanuts do not combine to form a high-quality protein in the way that grains and other legumes do.

Minimal Protein Requirements

To the extent that a person manages to circumvent the granola, cheese, and peanut butter pitfalls, he will probably do so by virtue of having understood precisely how much protein he needs and how to provide it more appropriately. The optimal amount of protein per day for an adult has been a matter of prolonged controversy. Some experts say protein is commonly taken in excess and that this may cause problems.[51,52] Others maintain that it is practically impossible to get too much.[53] Adele Davis, one of the pioneers of diet consciousness in twentieth-century America, advocated obtaining at least 90 grams of protein a day. Other authors have suggested that 30 grams is quite adequate,[52,54] and some studies have even indicated that under 10 grams might be sufficient in certain cases.[55] With such vastly different figures being mentioned, it's no wonder that many people feel confused about what the correct protein intake is for a normal adult.

Research on this question is complicated by the fact that there are a number of methods used to investigate protein needs in humans, all of them being somewhat awkward and none of them yielding unequivocal results.[nt.2] Nevertheless, in recent years a certain tentative consensus has been reached. The recommended dietary allowance (RDA) for protein in the U.S., based on World Health Organization guidelines,[56] is 0.8 grams of protein per kilogram of body weight per day. This translates into 45 to 55 grams of protein a day for a man who weighs 150 pounds, while the range for a 130-pound woman would be more like 40 to 45. We could say, then, that as a rule of thumb most adults would be amply supplied by a daily intake of 40 to 50 grams.

But protein requirements are not the same in every situation or for every person. As with any nutrient, there are a number of factors responsible for how much a given person should take in. First, there is the question of absorption. Protein that exits with the stool is of little benefit. Absorption depends on a huge variety of factors: the nature of the food, cooking techniques, how thoroughly the food is chewed, the concentration of digestive enzymes that it comes in contact with, and so on. Tough meat, fried and chewed poorly, is less likely to be well digested. If the person who ate the meal has a weak digestion and secretes unusually low concentrations of digestive juices, the absorption of the protein will be even further reduced. Even after protein is acted on by digestive enzymes, broken down, and passes through the intestinal wall into the bloodstream, there are differences in utilization. Some people use up more of it than others. So when we say that 40 to 50 grams of protein is enough for most people, questions may still arise in our mind. How many is most? What are the chances that I am an exception? If there are marked differences in individual needs, how likely am I to get adequate protein at this level?

In fact, the 40- to 50-gram guideline has been formulated with such differences in mind. Protein requirements, like most biological variations, tend to fall in a predictable pattern—what statisticians call a bell-shaped curve. Most people have moderate protein needs and hence fall near the middle of the curve. There are fewer and fewer cases of either extreme, that is, of very low or very high requirements at each end of the bell-shaped curve. RDAs for protein include adjustments for such variations as rate of absorption, and will cover 97% of the adult population. Actual individual needs probably range from about 27 grams to 55 grams a day for a 150-pound man, with only 1% or 2% of men requiring the upper figure.

In terms of common foods, 50 grams of protein may seem like a lot. A cup of milk supplies about 10 grams, an egg 6 or 8. If we relied solely on such so-called high-protein foods for our intake, we'd be in trouble: we'd have to eat a half dozen eggs a day or drink over a quart of milk. But other foods contain protein too, even though such foods may be predominantly carbohydrate. For example, a half cup of cooked legumes will contain nearly 8 grams of protein, close to what is found in an egg or a cup of milk. Of course, its amino acid makeup limits its value, unless it's combined with a grain.

But even the most clumsy efforts at combining proteins will usually yield a limiting amino acid that's better than 75% of the ideal, and the recommended allowance was adjusted to ensure adequate intake with a quality as low as that. A cup of rice will have about 4 grams of protein, and the beans and rice together will result in 12 grams of high-quality protein, more than that in a cup of milk or an egg. If most of our protein is of reasonably good quality, our requirement will probably be somewhat less than 40 to 50 grams a day.

A meal of rice and beans with a green vegetable, including milk

Protein Content of Vegetarian Foods (Average Servings)

Food	Amount	Calorie Content	Protein (grams)
Milk (2%)	1 cup	140	10
Low-fat cottage cheese	1/3 cup	40	8
Egg	1 (large)	80	7
Rice	1 cup	225	4
Beans	1/2 cup	100	8
Bread, whole-wheat	1 slice (c. 1 oz.)	65	3
Spinach (cooked)	2/3 cup	25	4
Broccoli	1 medium stalk	50	6
Collards	2/3 cup	40	5
Orange	1 (medium)	70	2
Raspberries	1 cup	85	2
Banana	1 (medium)	100	1

Source: U.S. Dept. of Agriculture: *Nutritive Value of American Foods.*[44]

products such as cottage cheese and yogurt to equal one cup of milk, and a slice of whole-grain bread, will provide 28 grams of good-quality protein, at an energy intake of only about 600 calories. If you use some butter on your bread and in cooking, add another 150 calories. Even 750 calories is only about a third of the usual daily intake. So if a person has satisfied more than half his protein needs in a single meal, while getting only a third of his calories, then he's not likely to end up protein deficient at the end of the day.

It is just such data that have led nutritionists experienced in computing nutrient intakes on well-balanced meatless diets to conclude that it is hard not to *exceed* protein allowances when caloric needs are met.[54] In other words, when whole foods are used, adequate protein intake is automatic. Because of this, a group of researchers studying protein nutrition at Harvard had trouble devising an experimental diet using plant foods that was low enough in protein to cause deficiency symptoms. They concluded: "It is difficult to obtain a mixed vegetable diet which will produce an appreciable loss of body nitrogen [protein] without resorting to high levels of sugar, jams, and jellies, and other essentially protein-free foods."[57]

Of course, that's exactly when the problems arise: when one throws in high-calorie, low-protein (or non-protein) foods, such as candies, pastries, chips and dips, and other foods rich in fats or sugars. Doing that will soon use up one's calorie quota for the day without meeting one's protein needs. To be adequate, such diets must be bolstered with high-protein foods like tofu, milk, eggs, fish, or even meat and poultry.[nt.12]

In affluent societies, where meat is consistently available and regularly included in meals, it comes to be relied on as the prime protein source. As dietary practices develop around this, the other items in the meal that accompany the meat tend to evolve in directions that complement a high-protein food and that capitalize on its presence. If one can count on the presence of animal foods for his protein needs, he can indulge his tastes for high-fat, high-sugar, and refined-flour treats. Therefore fried potatoes, white bread, oily salad dressing, and generous desserts have become the traditional accessories to the standard steak or chicken dinner.

The regular repetition of a customary diet is associated with the development of tastes and preferences that have their own compelling forcefulness. This becomes a major complication in the transition to a new protein source. As meat is phased out, the rest of the diet must begin to change too, or protein deficiency can become a serious problem. Though a diet based primarily on plant foods should easily satisfy protein needs, populations in the throes of dietary transition may not successfully use it to do so. Unless new eating habits are developed deliberately, on the basis of sound nutritional principles, they may fail to provide for sufficient protein and other nutrients. This liability is perhaps peculiar to situations wherein family and cultural influences have waned, massive change is in progress, and there are no coherent or consistent models available on which to base new eating habits.

Special Protein Requirements

Protein intakes should be higher for infants and children, who are growing and adding muscle bulk. Their diets should supply as much as 2 grams of protein per kilogram per day in the first few months of life, decreasing gradually to adult levels by the age of 18. Pregnancy also increases protein needs, which rise gradually through gestation to a peak of 6 grams of protein per kilogram per day near the end of term. This is almost 10 times the normal requirement. During nursing, the mother will still need an extra 50% more than the usual adult requirement.[56]

On the other hand, contrary to popular impression, there is no evidence that protein levels need to be elevated during periods of physical exertion—for example, in athletic training. The only exception to this is the need for a small amount of extra protein to develop new muscle tissue during intensive training.[56] Even that does not mean the percentage of protein in the food should be raised, for during athletic training one's caloric intake will generally increase, and unless it does so through the addition of sweets and greasy foods, protein intake will also increase as a result. The extra food eaten brings along more than enough additional protein to supply what is required for new muscle development.[58]

In fact, because of their increased caloric intake, athletes undergoing endurance training only needed to get 6.5% of their calories as protein,[58] though protein needs are ordinarily gauged at 8% to 9% of the energy intake of the diet. Intakes of protein on an average diet usually run close to 12% of calories,[56] so an ordinary selection of foods is likely to supply almost twice the amount of protein needed. In other words, the belief that the athlete needs to "beef up" his or her diet with extra protein-rich foods has not been backed up by scientific evidence.

Protein Supplementation for the Vegetarian Diet

There are other legitimate reasons for supplementing the diet with a moderate amount of protein-rich food. One of those has to do with the quality of the vegetables, grains, and beans available today. For example, although reference books on nutrition will list, without qualification, a single protein content for wheat, analyses have shown that the amount can vary widely. Wheat grown in Canada has more than half again as much protein as that grown in England.[59] Much of the difference has to do with the condition of the soils. When land becomes depleted, the nutrient content of crops grown on it falls. Although in the United States soils have not been farmed for as long as those in England, modern mechanized agriculture has accelerated erosion and taken its toll on America's farmlands. For example, it has been said that the protein content of wheat grown in Kansas fell about a third in a period of only 11 years.[60]

A few tablespoons of tofu or cottage cheese, or a sprinkling of small bits of fish or meat, is usually enough to accomplish adequate supplementation. It is interesting that in many, if not most, dietary traditions, when animal foods are used they are customarily limited to such modest amounts. One may not, however, be aware of this fact, since ethnic restaurants in affluent countries usually offer versions of these traditional dishes that depart from customary proportions, increasing the protein-rich and fat-rich animal foods.

Protein supplementation should not be exaggerated. It is important to recall that current experiments suggest that excess protein can be damaging to the kidneys.[61] Researchers also feel that high-protein diets may well contribute to the decline in kidney function that occurs as one grows older and that has been attributed to normal aging. Other studies suggest that diets high in animal protein increase one's risk of kidney stones[62] and gallstones.[63] Moreover, the extra ammonia that results from the breakdown of excess protein has even been thought to hasten cell proliferation and to contribute to the development of malignant growths.[64] There is also a good deal of evidence that diets high in animal protein interfere with proper calcium metabolism and can contribute to the development of osteoporosis, a problem of increasing proportions in developing countries.

CALCIUM, VITAMIN D, AND OSTEOPOROSIS

The vegetarian diet brings both assets and liabilities. Though its protein content turns out, as we have seen, not to be the problem that is often expected, there are some other, more serious, concerns. For example, getting adequate vitamin D and zinc requires attention, and we will look at these nutrients and how to satisfy one's requirements for them later in this chapter. But the meatless diet has some pleasant surprises in store for us, too. One of the most welcome of these is its potential for preventing the extensive demineralization of the bones that occurs in osteoporosis. The recent recognition of the prevalence of this disease has been followed by a hasty attempt to deal with it through taking calcium supplements. We will look at the underlying principles of the demineralization process and at how diet, along with moderate exercise, can provide a better way to prevent development of this common, crippling disease.

What Is Osteoporosis?

Osteoporosis is a loss of minerals from the bones, a process that leaves them porous and fragile so that they are easily fractured. Approximately half the women over 50 in the U.S.

develop osteoporosis to some degree and half of those with the disease suffer fractures as a result. Broken hips are the most common, but compression fractures of the vertebrae are not unusual and are responsible for the humped back and loss in height experienced by those who have the disease.

Osteoporosis has become so prevalent that it's sometimes considered a normal part of the aging process. It isn't. In one survey more than one third of men and one fifth of women aged 55 to 64 lost little or no bone at all during an 11-year period.[65] Though why some people are more susceptible than others is not entirely clear, there are a number of well-established risk factors:

1. Calcium absorption. Older people often lose a certain percentage of their capacity to absorb nutrients. This includes calcium.
2. Vitamin D levels. Vitamin D is necessary for calcium absorption to occur. Older people often get too little sunshine and may have no alternate source of vitamin D.[66] In such cases, taking vitamin D slows bone loss.[67]
3. Older people often exercise less. Exercise is a powerful stimulation of bone mineralization. People over 50 who did about a half hour of running daily had bone density 40% higher than a comparable group who exercised little.[68]
4. Decreased estrogen/testosterone. The sex hormones are major promoters of the deposition of minerals in the bones. A woman's estrogen levels drop off suddenly at menopause. A man's testosterone levels decrease much more gradually. Thus, postmenopausal women are particularly susceptible to osteoporosis.[69]
5. Reduction of kidney function with aging averages about 30%. This undermines one's ability to filter selectively, and calcium that should be retained is lost through the urine.
6. Peak bone mass: Bones reach their maximal strength and weight at about age 30. A greater peak bone mass means one is less likely to demineralize the bones to the point of danger later in life. White men and black people of both sexes have a higher average peak bone mass than white women, and it is thought that this is one of the reasons they have less osteoporosis as they grow older. Children and adolescents who have poor diets will

have a lower peak bone mass at age 30 and will be especially vulnerable to osteoporosis later.[70] Preventing the disease, then, is something that should start very early in life. It is important to understand the principles of mineral nutrition so that they can be applied from childhood onwards.

How Much Calcium?

Calcium affects not only the health of the bones and teeth, but also the ability of the muscles to contract properly, and even the condition of the nervous system. With inadequate calcium the bones will demineralize, the muscles will go into spasm, and the nervous system will become irritable and hypersensitive. Though such extreme symptoms of calcium deficiency are rare, milder versions may be common. Vague irritability or intermittent leg cramps in children or older people may not be recognized as being related to insufficient calcium.

The official recommended daily allowance (RDA) of calcium by the Food and Nutrition Board is 800 milligrams a day (the amount in three cups of milk) for both adults and children under 10, who need much more calcium per pound of body weight, since they are actively building bones and teeth. During the rapid growth that occurs from ages 10 to 18, even more—1,200 milligrams a day—is recommended.[71] A recent survey[72] showed that 80% to 85% of adult females and 50% to 65% of adult males had calcium intakes below the recommended 800 milligrams a day. About half the children under 10 get less than the RDA, and adolescents do even worse, with 60% of adolescent boys and 85% of girls getting less than the RDA.[72] A large percentage of adolescent girls are thus thought to be presently creating a vulnerability to osteoporosis when they grow older.

The situation among the elderly only compounds the risk. Only about a third of people over 65 get 800 milligrams of calcium a day,[73] and this at precisely the time when their needs are going up due to a decreasing ability to absorb the mineral from their food[74] and an increased tendency to decalcification of the bones.

If inadequate dietary levels are as common as these figures suggest, calcium supplementation on a national scale would seem imperative. In fact, many food processors are now voluntarily fortifying their products with calcium, though this practice is not mandatory as it is with other nutrients like iron or thiamin. But whether this is a good idea or not is unclear. Dietary requirements for calcium are still a matter of some debate. The World Health Organization set an allowance of barely more than half that accepted in the U.S., 400 to 500 milligrams per day.[75]

The requirement for calcium is established, as it is for other nutrients, through balance studies: calcium intake and calcium output are measured. As long as there is no net loss, a person is assumed to be getting enough calcium in the diet. Studies done in a number of countries have shown that calcium balance can often be maintained on intakes as low as 200 to 300 milligrams a day.[75]

By these standards, Americans are getting more than ample calcium. But if that's true, then why is osteoporosis epidemic? To answer that question, we will need to probe a bit deeper into some of the more important factors that influence calcium absorption and metabolism.

Vitamin D and Calcium Absorption

Not all the calcium consumed manages to find its way from the food into the body's tissues. Only 20% to 30% is ordinarily absorbed, even in young, healthy adults, and absorptive capacity usually declines through life. How much calcium is absorbed depends to a great extent on how much vitamin D is present.

Vitamin D is formed in the skin during exposure to sunlight. It then goes through several additional steps inside the body, resulting in its eventual transformation into a potent promoter of calcium absorption. Without vitamin D, the calcium in food is of little use, since it will pass through the intestinal tract unassimilated, and exit with the feces. In addition to the critical role it plays in getting calcium into the body, vitamin D also makes it possible for minerals to be removed from one part of the bone so they can be redeposited in another, thus reshaping the contours of the bone. This is a process that is particularly important in childhood and youth, when bones are growing, but continues to some extent throughout life. Therefore, even though we may think of vitamin

D as creating strong bones, the effect of vitamin D on the bone is a resorptive one. Whereas too little of it will cause the bones to be misshapen, too much can cause them to be demineralized.[nt.13]

The skeletal deformities that result from vitamin D deficiency are called rickets. This disease is common among children who fail to get sufficient vitamin D in the diet or who don't get enough sunshine, which forms vitamin D in the skin. It was a widespread problem in England at the time of the Industrial Revolution, when smoke and smog so obscured the sun that many children developed disfiguring cases of the disease. The disease has also been reported recently in England and America among emigrants from Southeast Asia, whose diets contain little vitamin D and who are accustomed to relying on the intense sunshine of their native climates for it. Rickets is also being seen with increasing frequency in the U.S. among vegetarian children who do not take dairy products and who live in colder climates where exposure to sunshine is minimal. For example, 32 children in Boston, following a Japanese-influenced vegetarian diet with no dairy products, eggs, or fish, were studied carefully. They were getting an average of 33 International Units (IU) a day, less than one tenth of the 400 IU that is recommended. Daily intakes ranged from zero to 270 IU.[80] The barest minimum of vitamin D necessary to ensure the absorption of enough calcium to maintain life is thought to be somewhere between 40 and 100 IU a day; 100 IU is said to prevent rickets, though 400 IU is considered necessary to promote better calcium absorption and allow some increase in growth rate.[81] Not only did the children in Boston have low intakes of vitamin D, but half also had elevated levels of an enzyme, alkaline phosphatase,[80] that is usually taken as an indicator that bone is being broken down faster than it's being built up.

The problem of an adequate vitamin D supply is solved when the vegetarian diet includes milk or fish. Fish oils, especially fish liver oils, are rich in vitamin D. Though milk itself is thought to be relatively low, milk in the United States contains an additive from plant sources called ergosterol. After being irradiated, the molecular structure of this substance is active in those reactions that require vitamin D. A quart of fortified milk supplies about 400 IU of vitamin D; boiling or cooking with the milk will not destroy it to any significant extent.[81]

For those who do not take milk or fish, vitamin D is easily available in capsules, but the total daily intake should be kept within the range of 300 to 500 IU (10 milligrams) for both children and adults. Taking more "to be safe" is not wise, nor is it safe, because of the adverse effects of excess vitamin D.[nt.13]

Recently it has become customary for vitamin D to be added to animal feeds, presumably to encourage growth. As a result, animal fats are likely to contain high concentrations of the vitamin. Research suggests that the average American may currently be consuming as much as 2,400 IU of vitamin D a day,[76,82] partly from the fat of beef and chicken and partly from multivitamin and mineral supplements and fortified foods such as white flour, bread, and breakfast cereals. Though milk may supply needed vitamin D for the person whose diet contains no meat or common fortified foods, it may not be desirable for the average meat-eater, who already runs the risk of getting too much vitamin D.

Regulating Vitamin D Intake

If you still use meat, poultry, and fish as well as milk and commercial breads and cereals, don't take vitamin D supplements. Read labels and tally your intake. Try to stay near 400 IU.

If you use all-natural whole foods, consume a pint of milk a day, and get some sunshine, you're probably OK. If not, you may need to take a vitamin D supplement.

There are other factors besides a deficiency of vitamin D that can decrease absorption of calcium. As is true in the case of other minerals, such as iron, the percentage of dietary calcium that is normally absorbed can be decreased by the presence of certain calcium-binding substances found in plant foods. One might conclude that vegetarians, then, would be especially prone to calcium deficiency. This was long assumed to be the case, though as we shall see the truth turns out to be nearly the opposite.

Phytic Acid

As early as 1925 British nutritionists raised puppies (who are carnivores) on bread and found that although they grew rapidly, their bones were soft and malformed. The puppies were affected more when whole-wheat bread was used, and the result with oatmeal was even worse. The anticalcifying factor in whole grains was eventually identified and called phytic acid. It was found to form a complex with calcium that was not absorbed. Later, experiments showed that in humans, too, less calcium is absorbed from brown bread than white, and this strengthened the case against phytates. So when war rationing struck Britain and the use of brown bread was mandated to stretch grain supplies, calcium was added to cover the losses expected to occur due to the bran in the whole-meal bread.

Since that time, however, ideas have changed. It was found that part of the phytic acid can be split apart by an enzyme—phytase—active in wheat and rye during the rising of bread. This reduces the binding of calcium. Oats contain very little phytase (however, oats are not generally used to make raised bread). This may account for their producing the most severe rickets in the puppy experiment.

On the basis of such reasoning it was predicted that Scotland, where oatmeal is a hallowed tradition, would be grievously plagued with rickets. No such prevalence of the disease was evident, however, and the Scots' confidence in their oatmeal was vindicated when experiments on Scottish volunteers showed that the phytates from the grain were broken down in the intestinal tract of those accustomed to the regular consumption of oatmeal.[83] Later studies have confirmed that the tendency of phytic acid to capture calcium and carry it away is real enough, but that the human intestinal tract can produce phytase of its own, which enables it to break down phytic acid and free the calcium bound to it.[84] The ability to produce such phytase is thought to be developed in response to the regular consumption of high-phytate foods such as whole grains.[83]

Oxalic Acid

Oxalic acid is another component of vegetable foods that has often been accused of binding minerals such as calcium and preventing their absorption. In most cases the effect of oxalic acid in vegetables is probably negligible.[83] Some leafy vegetables, such as spinach and chard, that contain high levels of oxalic acid also contain respectable amounts of calcium, but the calcium is not well utilized unless the action of the oxalic acid can somehow be blocked. The addition of rice to the meals that include spinach or chard has been found to accomplish this and, as a result, to allow the proper utilization of the calcium in such vegetables. Other grains were not helpful in this way.[85]

Since vegetarian diets rely on grain/legume combinations and often include a bean and rice base, leafy vegetables such as chard and spinach may often function as significant sources of calcium after all. In any case, other leafy greens, such as collards, kale, or mustard greens, which do not contain significant amounts of oxalic acid and are richer in calcium anyway, remain superb sources of it (see table on p. 121).

Fiber

Besides phytates and oxalates, the fiber found in whole plant foods can also bind calcium and carry it out of the body. Cellulose, one of the coarser parts of vegetable fiber, found in peels and stalks as well as in bran, has been shown to block calcium absorption,[nt. 14] whereas the softer gelatinous fiber (pectin) found in the interiors of fruits and vegetables does not appear to inhibit its uptake.[86]

Bran may be particularly problematic: it contains both cellulose and phytates. Bran given for six weeks to elderly persons to relieve constipation lowered calcium levels in the blood.[87]

On the other hand, the primary component of fiber responsible for calcium binding has been found to be digested by bacteria in the colon. From there the mineral can be absorbed, and a person's capacity to do so is thought to gradually increase as he adjusts to a higher-fiber diet.[88] It would appear then that a person who has slowly and systematically adopted a vegetarian diet, allowing ample time for adjustment, will have little trouble with calcium absorption as long as he regularly consumes milk

Calcium Content of Foods

Food	Amount	Calcium (mg)
Milk (2%)	1 cup	350
Cheese, cheddar	1 oz slice	215
Cheese, cottage	3 oz (c. 1/2 cup)	80
Tofu	4 oz	150
Eggs	1 (large)	25
Chicken	4 oz (2 pieces)	10
Hamburger	3 oz patty	10
Bread, whole-wheat	1 slice (c. 1 oz)	25
Collards*	2/3 cup	320
Kale	2/3 cup	180
Mustard greens*	2/3 cup	170
Spinach*	2/3 cup	110
Swiss chard*	2/3 cup	85
Cabbage*	2/3 cup	45
Broccoli	1 medium stalk	158
Snap beans*	2/3 cup	45
Rice	1 cup	20
Kidney beans (cooked)	1/3 cup	20
Orange	1 (medium)	10

*Cooked in own broth until water evaporates (not drained); see p. 130.

Source: U.S. Dept. of Agriculture: *Nutritive Value of American Foods.*[44]

products or green leafy vegetables with his rice and bean combinations, generally avoids eating peelings, stems, and stalks, and refrains from lacing his food with bran.

Vegetarians Have Stronger Bones

That calcium absorption from plant foods is not seriously impaired is indicated by the fact that vegetarians have strong bones and that, even in later years, they tend to stay that way. At least two thorough studies have shown that vegetarians who consume milk do not lose bone mass as fast as their meat-eating counterparts[89,90] (see figure below). Although some research has failed to confirm this difference in men,[91] all studies agree that it is present in women, becoming especially striking after menopause. That is, among postmenopausal women—precisely that segment of the population most at risk for osteoporosis—those who are vegetarian have markedly less bone loss than those who eat meat.

Decalcification of the Bones in Women[nt.15]

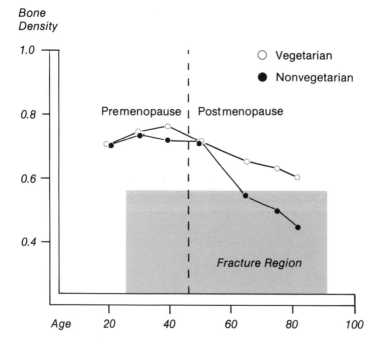

Bone Density as Related to Meat Consumption in Women Ages 70-79 in Three Populations[nt.15]

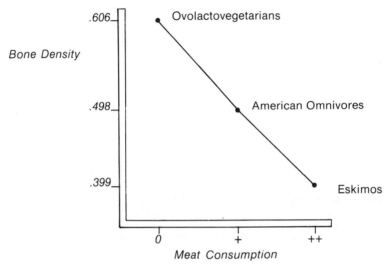

Sources: Marsh et al: *Cortical Bone Density.*[90] Mazess & Mather: *Bone Mineral Content.*[92]

Moreover, among vegetarians the bone loss slows or stops after about age 70, whereas in meat-eaters it continues.[89] This would suggest that vegetarians, as they reach their 70s and 80s, should have fewer hip fractures and compressed vertebrae.

At the other end of the spectrum, those who consume lots of meat present a very different picture. The Eskimos are an example. They must depend to a great extend on animal foods for their sustenance. Caribou, sea mammals, fish, and birds are their basic staples. As a result their diet is unusually high in meat and fat, and they provide an opportunity to observe the effects of such a diet on bone metabolism. Surveys have shown that in Eskimos the onset of bone loss begins in the late 30s—10 to 20 years earlier than in the average American. The decreased density of the bones is associated with an increased frequency of fractures and tooth loss. Since the Arctic populations studied were quite active and take plenty of marine foods that are rich in vitamin D, researchers have attributed their accelerated bone loss to their high meat intake.[92]

What emerges, then, from a comparison of the typical picture of osteoporosis in elderly American women with those who eat no meat, on the one hand, and with those who eat extremely large amounts of meat, on the other, is a clear correlation between meat-eating and bone loss. The more meat eaten, the more the bones are demineralized.

The relative freedom from osteoporosis enjoyed by vegetarians poses some interesting questions that medical science will need to ponder as it works to conquer this increasingly prevalent disease: Why would vegetarians be less susceptible? What effects do animal foods have? Are meat and poultry different from dairy products? Though all the answers aren't in yet, some of the pieces of the puzzle are already falling into place.

It is known, for example, that high levels of fat in the diet interfere with calcium absorption. Fatty acids tend to react with calcium ions, forming insoluble soaps that exit with the feces. Saturated, long-chain fatty acids such as those found in the fat of beef are particularly likely to do so. Medium-chain and short-chain fatty acids, which are more common in butterfat, are less likely to do so.[93] In fact, it has been suggested that butter facilitates absorption of the substantial amounts of calcium found in milk.[94] There are other reasons, too, why milk should prove to be a great asset. Milk sugar, lactose, has its own promoting effect on calcium absorption,[83] and the balance of minerals in milk is especially conducive to mineralizing the bones, as we shall see later. Research has confirmed that dairy products have a beneficial effect on the bones[95] that is superior to that of calcium supplements.

Another possible reason why vegetarians have less osteoporosis is that meat diets are usually higher in protein,[96] and protein intakes in the same range as those typical of meat-eaters increase the loss of calcium through the urine.[97] It is thought that the additional protein residues increase the rate of filtration through the kidney, pulling along more calcium.

Moreover, as mentioned in the previous chapter, the residues that result from both the protein and the fat of meat and poultry are acidic. A diet that shifts body chemistry in an acidic direction is thought by some researchers to be another, independent, factor that causes calcium loss[nt.16] and contributes to the development of osteoporosis.[90,98,99] This may well be an additional reason why elderly vegetarians have stronger bones.

Calcium/Phosphorus Ratios

Animal products usually contain much more phosphorus than calcium. At least that is true of meat, poultry, and most fish, though dairy products are the opposite. It has long been known that an excess of phosphorus in the diet can demineralize the bones. But only recently has it become clear exactly how this happens.

It is critical for the welfare of such organs as the heart and brain that calcium levels in the blood be kept constant. If there is an increase or decrease, immediate steps are taken to correct this. This regulation is accomplished by a hormone that comes from tiny glands located on each side of the thyroid. These are the parathyroid glands, and the hormone is parathyroid hormone— often shortened to parathormone, or PTH. As soon as blood levels of calcium begin to fall, PTH is secreted and pulls calcium into the blood by mobilizing it from the bones. Thus bone serves as a sort of reservoir for calcium, which can be drawn on in emergencies to maintain calcium availability for vital tissues.

Parathormone also throws several other switches that help restore blood calcium. It causes the kidneys to hang on to calcium rather than letting it go out with the urine, and it increases the intestinal absorption of calcium by activating vitamin D. In other words, PTH is the master regulator of calcium metabolism (see figure on p. 127). It responds instantaneously to the least drop in calcium levels, quickly setting them right.

One of the most common events that lower levels of calcium and thereby trigger PTH release is an influx into the bloodstream of extra phosphorus. If a meal is richer in phosphorus than in calcium, calcium levels are driven downward for a few hours as the unbalanced phosphates reach the blood.[101] During this time, due to the dip in calcium levels, the parathyroid glands come to the rescue, putting out more parathormone. PTH not only mobilizes calcium from the bone and stops it from leaving through the kidneys, it also forces the offending phosphates out of the bloodstream and into the urine. So PTH manages to get rid of phosphorus while holding on to calcium.

Paradoxically, then, while a high-phosphate meal is causing a net calcium gain for the body as a whole, it is also resulting in calcium loss from the bone.[100, 102] If the body as a whole is gaining calcium while the bones are losing it, then where does it go? It isn't allowed to build up in the blood. Yet the tendency of PTH to acquire and to hold on to calcium creates a kind of pressure. Due to this force, the retained calcium is shunted into the extracellular fluid. It's as though the calcium gained were being squeezed out of the bones and the blood into the soft tissues of the body.

But too much calcium is as much of a problem as too little. The cells normally keep levels of calcium inside themselves at less than a thousandth of what is outside. This is necessary because high concentrations of calcium inside will react with vital molecules such as ATP, creating insoluble compounds that no longer function properly.[103] It has been suggested that a rise in calcium levels inside the cells is one of the basic events involved in many chronic diseases and that it may be a fundamental cause of cell death and of the tissue deterioration that we call aging.[104-5, nt. 17]

To the extent that the cells succeed in keeping the calcium that was squeezed into the tissues by PTH outside of themselves, the calcium will usually accumulate in nooks and crannies as mineral deposits. Favorite, relatively harmless, spots for depositing it are joint spaces and arterial walls, where it helps form osteoarthritic bone spurs and calcified atherosclerotic plaques.[100] Though sweeping it under the rug in this fashion is at least a short-term solution, serious mechanical obstruction will eventually develop.

Estrogen and Bone Disease

Bone is alive and metabolically active. There's a constant tug-of-war going on between those forces acting to deposit minerals and those acting to reabsorb them from the bone. Which

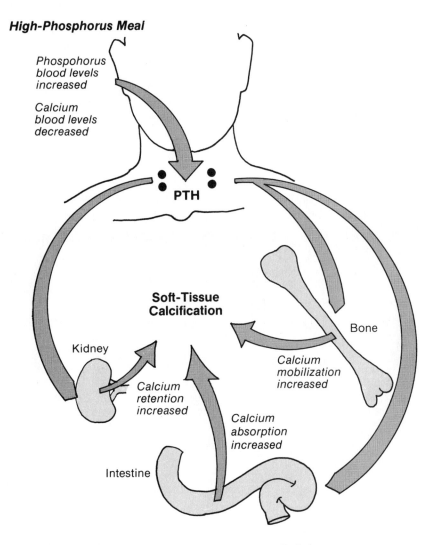

Effect of Parathyroid Hormone (PTH) on Calcium Metabolism:
How High-Phosphorus Meals Trigger PTH Release, Causing Bone Loss and Soft-Tissue Calcification

Source: Schaafsma: *Influence of Dietary Calcium.*[100]

side prevails will determine whether the bones get gradually softer and more fragile or stronger and more dense. When mobilization is stimulated by PTH it will exceed deposition unless deposition is also quite vigorous.

Among the most important of the promoters of bone deposition are estrogen and testosterone. In women past menopause, whose estrogen levels are low, the stage is set for a diet higher in phosphates than in calcium—because of such a diet's repeated stimulation of PTH release—to gradually, over a period of time, demineralize the bones. One might picture each successive surge of unbalanced phosphates that enters the blood after a calcium-poor, phosphorus-rich meal as washing through the bones and carrying minerals away, much as the successive waves of the rising tide wash sand from a beach.

Recent estimates put the average calcium/phosphorus ratio in

Calcium/Phosphorus Ratios of Common Foods

Ca:P (High Ca)		1:1		Ca:P (High P)
green leafy vegetables 2.5:1 to 6:1	dairy products* 1.4:1	non-leafy green vegetables	grains and beans 1:2 to 1:5	meat, poultry, fish 1:15+
herbs and spices 2:1 to 28:1			Eggs 1:3	nutr. yeast 1:9
carob powder 4:1	green beans and broccoli 1.4:1		asparagus 1:2	soft drinks 1:∞**
maple syrup 13:1†		fresh fruits		wheat bran 1:10
	oranges and pineapples 2:1	apples 1:1.6	bananas 1:3	

Items in bold are those which are calculated (by virtue of their mineral content and volume of use) to have the most significant impact on calcium metabolism when included in the diet in the usual amounts.

*Except cottage cheese, which is 1:2.

**Soft drinks vary in their mineral content—most have no calcium but moderate to high levels of phosphorous.

†Although maple syrup has a good ratio of calcium to phosphorus, it is high in sugar and should not be used in large quantities.

Source: U.S. Dept. of Agriculture: *Nutritive Value of American Foods.*[44]

the American diet at about 1:1.5. The ideal ratio of calcium to phosphorus in the diet is usually considered to be 1:1, though even more calcium may be advantageous.[102] In the strongly meat-oriented diet, the phosphorus content is much higher than that of calcium, because phosphorus is naturally more abundant in most of the major foodstuffs used. Meat, poultry, and fish supply 15 to 20 times as much phosphorus as calcium, while eggs, grains, nuts, and legumes provide about twice as much.

Only milk, unprocessed cheeses, and green leafy vegetables contain substantially more calcium than phosphorus,[106] though a number of other green vegetables and certain fruits also have a favorable ratio (see chart on p. 128). We must rely on adequate intakes of these foods to rectify the imbalances created by foods higher in phosphorus. With this principle in mind, dishes such as those based on leafy greens become quite important, and it is critical to learn how to prepare them in a way that makes them both digestible and appetizing.

Significant quantities of phosphates may also come into the current American diet by way of additives. Many of the conditioners and preservatives used in foods are phosphates. Sodium phosphate, pyrophosphate, and monohydrogen phosphate are a few common ones likely to be listed on the labels of foods and beverages. Although these additives are considered relatively nontoxic, the level of them in the diet is thought to be increasing sufficiently to disturb the calcium/phosphorus ratio significantly.[101-2] This is especially likely in the context of a high-meat diet, where calcium/phosphorus ratios are already skewed. Vitamin and mineral supplements may also contain substantial amounts of phosphorus, since it is intentionally added so that all the essential minerals will be included.

If calcium/phosphorus ratios are kept reasonable, then it may not be not so important whether calcium intakes are high or merely moderate. On a healthful, low-phosphorus, vegetarian diet a calcium intake of 500 to 600 milligrams may be quite sufficient. With the basic principles of bone metabolism understood, and with the calcium and phosphorus contents of foods in mind, one should be able to devise a well-balanced vegetarian diet that is maximally effective in preventing osteoporosis.

How to Use Leafy Greens

1. Availability varies. Try what you can find.
2. Wash each leaf thoroughly to remove grit.
3. Remove stems, discard discolored leaves.
4. Chop to speed cooking. Parboil if bitter or strong.
5. Season simply with butter and salt or make flavor more robust with fried onions and spices (see discussion of flavor bases on pp. 138-41).
6. Cook until tender (20 to 40 minutes). Pressure cook tough greens.
7. Do not drain; serve in own broth if there is any.
8. Add milk near end of cooking to subdue strong or acid flavors.

Other vegetables may be cooked along with the greens, or tofu may be added near the end. Paneer (see recipe on p. 210) is especially useful and is cubed and added 5 to 10 minutes before the vegetable is done.[nt.18]

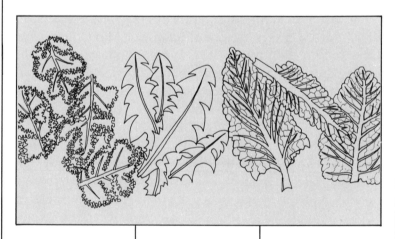

collards	chard	amaranth
mustard greens	escarole	turnip greens
spinach	broccoli rabe	dandelion greens
New Zealand	kale	osome
spinach	beet tops	tatsoi
lamb's-quarters		

Other Minerals

A vegetarian diet may also be of help in preventing osteoporosis for other reasons besides its beneficial effects on calcium metabolism. Though it is present in the largest amounts, calcium is only one of the minerals needed by the bones. Others, such as magnesium, silicon, fluorine, and manganese, are equally necessary for normal mineralization. Magnesium is needed in quantities that may be close to those of calcium. Others need be present in only tiny amounts.

Manganese is a case in point. Though only traces of it are necessary, rats that get in the diet less than the small amounts normally present develop porous bones similar to those seen in osteoporotic patients. When a research team examined blood and bone samples from 14 women with advanced osteoporosis and compared them with those of age-matched women without the disease, the only statistically significant difference between the two was in levels of manganese. Blood manganese in the women with osteoporosis was only one fourth that in the other group.[108] Other studies suggest that calcium supplements may inhibit manganese absorption, though milk as a source of calcium does not.[109]

Summing Up:
How to Prevent Osteoporosis

1. Exercise regularly.
2. Minimize animal foods—except dairy products, which are very beneficial.
3. Maintain vitamin D intakes near 400 IU a day.
4. Watch calcium/phosphorus ratios of frequently used foods; get lots of those with a high ratio (e.g., cooked leafy green vegetables).
5. Use calcium supplements on a limited basis and only if necessary.
6. Be sure intake of other minerals—such as magnesium and the trace minerals—is adequate. (See below.)

TRACE MINERALS AND THE SECRETS
OF SEASONING

Manganese is only one of a number of minerals found in tissues of the body in much smaller amounts than are calcium, magnesium, or iron. They are generally called trace minerals, and their importance is only just beginning to be appreciated. Until recent decades the presence of these minerals in the body and in foods was thought to be accidental. The discovery of small amounts of copper, zinc, or manganese in the ash of burned plant and animal tissue was attributed to contamination. As our research methods have become more sophisticated, however, it has been discovered that these tiny amounts of minerals are in fact critical to the proper functioning of the body. Their most dramatic role is as strategic components of enzymes.

Every metabolic reaction in the body depends on the presence of an enzyme to make it move along at the speed necessary to sustain life processes. Enzymes are huge protein molecules with slots or grooves in them where the smaller molecules that they are acting on can fit, much as a key would fit into a lock. When the smaller compounds to be processed slide into the slots of the enzyme molecules, they are brought into contact with a single atom of one of the trace minerals, such as zinc or copper. In some little-understood fashion, this contact triggers the desired reaction. The orchestration of the metabolic reactions going on in all the tissues is based on the presence of adequate quantities of the appropriate enzymes at each site. If an enzyme is deficient, the metabolic processes related to it will be slowed down and the overall functioning of the body will suffer. The end result of such a deficiency can range all the way from the kind of breakdown in specific tissues that we call disease to a general sense of lethargy, a lack of energy, and a clouded consciousness.

Enzymes can be manufactured in adequate quantities only if the trace minerals that are necessary for their construction are present in adequate amounts. With the increasing availability of precise diagnostic tools and the use of routine tests of trace element status, it is becoming obvious that deficiencies are common. They are due to a decrease of trace minerals like zinc, manganese, and selenium in our food supplies. Processed foods are lower in minerals than are foods that are whole and unaltered. For example, bread made from white flour has only about one fourth the zinc that whole wheat has. But even whole wheat can vary in mineral content, depending on the soil in which it was grown. Faulty agricultural practices that are now commonplace have progressively depleted the soil of its mineral content,[110-11] with the result that the plants grown on that soil are deficient.

Trace Mineral Content of Plants and Soils

The ultimate outcome of these trends is an increasing incidence of disorders that are recognized as being related to trace mineral deficiencies.[112] Selenium deficiencies have been reported to be associated with a greater risk of both heart disease and cancer,[113-17] and a recent study revealed a troubling association between birth defects and low manganese levels in both infants and their mothers.[118]

Though it seems particularly important before and during pregnancy to ensure adequate stores of trace minerals, it is important for everyone. The tissues of animals that are used as food contain enzymes, if not in optimal quantities at least in a quantity sufficient to sustain life. Otherwise the livestock from which it came would not have survived to the age of slaughter. This means that red meat and fowl, although not ideal, are at least dependable sources of some moderate amounts of trace minerals.

Plants, by contrast, do not require for their functioning some of the trace minerals that animals and humans require. Therefore plants grown on poor soil may reach maturity and be harvested without having taken up certain of the trace minerals that may be important to humans. This is true of iodine, for example. Moreover, as was the case with iron and calcium, the phytic acid and fiber that are present in plant foods have caused concern among nutritionists about the ability to absorb adequate trace minerals from them.[119]

A survey of vegetarians in Sweden showed their blood levels of selenium to be lower than those of meat-eaters.[120] But Scandinavian soils are notoriously low in selenium, a fact that has led

Finland to institute a policy of fortifying common foodstuffs with the mineral. Studies done in North America have come up with different results. A recent survey of 36 postmenopausal vegetarian women compared their mineral levels with those of meat-eaters. Copper and selenium status of the long-term vegetarians was comparable to that of the meat-eaters "despite the high intake of fiber in the vegetarian group." Moreover, manganese was higher— almost twice as high—in the vegetarians.[121] It would seem, then, that plant foods are an adequate source of some of the trace minerals. But there is at least one important exception, and that is zinc.

Zinc Deficiency in Vegetarians

When several hundred apparently normal persons of various ages from upper-income and middle-income families in Denver were surveyed, 10 boys from ages 4 to 13 were found to have exceptionally low zinc levels. On further investigation, it was found that all but 1 of these boys were well under normal height or weight for their age—smaller than 90% of their peers. Most of them were described by their families as having a poor appetite. Taste acuity tests showed their sense of taste was impaired.

After the boys were given small amounts of zinc for a few months, taste-test scores returned to normal, appetites improved, and 4 of them showed an acceleration in growth. When the mothers of the boys were interviewed, they reported that their sons had eaten a reasonable amount of food during the time when they had developed the deficiency, but that they had generally eaten only very small servings of meat, about one ounce a day, even though more was available.[122] Meat, poultry, and fish are by far the richest sources of zinc. Although some vegetable foods contain substantial amounts of it, fiber and phytates appear to carry much of this out of the body. Though manganese and copper are well absorbed from plant foods, zinc, like iron or calcium, seems more problematic, and nutritionists have expressed concern over the availability of zinc in the vegetarian diet.

There are research studies that indicate this concern may well be justified. For example, when a group of students were put on a vegetarian diet for three weeks, their tissue levels of zinc dropped and they responded to physiological tests in a way that suggested they had developed a mild zinc deficiency.[119]

But three weeks isn't long. We know that in the case of other minerals such as calcium some adaptation to the presence of fiber and phytates occurs and that, over time, absorption improves. So the research team looked next at a group of 79 persons that had been vegetarian for a year or longer. They found that their body levels of zinc were also low, despite the fact that they had been on the vegetarian diet for long periods of time.[96]

This is different from what we have seen in the case of calcium and perhaps iron, where adaptation seems to take place, and phytates and fiber seem to lose their tendency to interfere with mineral absorption. Why would zinc be different? The answer may lie in the fact that the enzyme that is developed to break down phytates, intestinal phytase, is itself zinc-dependent. Zinc is needed for the manufacture of phytase, and when zinc is deficient the enzyme cannot be produced in adequate amounts.[84] Less phytase means more phytate to interfere with the absorption of zinc, which in turn results in more severe zinc depletion, and still less phytase.

Once a zinc deficiency is established, it's obviously difficult to climb out of it—even with adequate zinc intake—as long as one's diet is rich in whole grains, which contain so much phytic acid. Once phytase production has been started, and zinc can be released from phytate and absorbed, handling a vegetarian diet is possible. But if a person's zinc stores are depleted during the transition phase, he won't be able to increase his output of phytase and adjust to the new diet. For such reasons, zinc supplements may be necessary during the time when one is changing over to a vegetarian diet.

Though the transition period is always tricky and is a time when developing zinc deficiency is especially likely, this risk is even higher if one starts out borderline. There is evidence, such as low zinc levels in patients with retarded wound-healing,[111] indicating that a significant percentage of the general, nonvegetarian population suffers from marginal zinc status.[111, 123-24] Girls and young women seem to have substandard intakes most often,[125-26] though men and boys, who tend to eat more animal foods, may become deficient despite their larger intakes, since the normal development and functioning of the male reproductive system requires a substantial intake of zinc. This is thought to be why it is mostly boys who have been found to be undersize as a result of zinc deficiency. In adult males, zinc deficiency can contribute to sterility and impotence.[124]

But zinc nutrition for pregnant and nursing women is perhaps of most serious concern, since the infant must draw its supply of zinc from the mother. Maternal zinc deprivation in experimental animals has produced offspring with learning disabilities[127] and abnormalities in the chemistry and structure of the brain, especially that part that is related to emotions.[128-29, nt.19] There is also evidence that zinc deficiency during pregnancy can lead to later impairment of immune function.

Low zinc later in life may also lead to a number of symptoms of immune deficiency[131] as well as impairment of the capacity to heal quickly. Inadequate tissue repair has been suspected of playing a role in the earliest stages of the development of atherosclerosis, where failure to heal properly some form of injury to the arterial lining may set the stage for plaque formation.[124]

If one does decide to take zinc supplements while adjusting to a vegetarian diet, 15 to 20 milligrams a day should be sufficient, since the recommended daily intake is only 15. Since absorption is only partial on any diet, this amount would not be excessive, especially when fiber and phytate levels are substantial.

In fact, zinc is one of the nutrients with the largest margin of safety. One would have to take well over 100 milligrams a day to cause any toxicity. But at even moderate doses zinc can compete with copper for absorption or utilization. Since vegetarian diets tend to be relatively rich in copper, this is not likely to be a problem. However, zinc can also interfere with selenium utilization, and though selenium too, as we have seen, is generally ample in vegetarian diets, zinc doses should be kept at reasonable levels for this reason. Though one may resort to supplements as a

Zinc Checklist

1. Keep fiber intake moderate.
2. Include tofu, beans, seeds, and nuts in your diet.
3. Watch for signs of zinc deficiency: white spots on nails, slow wound healing, poor resistance to infections, acne.
4. Consider supplementation—especially during transition phase.

temporary measure, in the meantime one should be developing the ability to plan and prepare meatless meals that are adequate in minerals such as zinc.

Besides milk and eggs, the nonmeat foods richest in zinc are beans, tofu, seeds, nuts, and hard cheeses. Of the lactovegetarians studied, men had higher intakes of zinc than women because they ate more of these foods.[132] The women tended to subsist on salads and fruits with much lower levels of a number of important nutrients, including zinc.[nt.20] The lowest zinc levels were seen in vegetarians who took no milk or eggs. Their fiber intake was much higher and their zinc intake lower than the lactovegetarians.[96]

Studies done on subjects who are more knowledgeable about the principles of nutrition and cooking indicate that they are less likely to become zinc deficient.[134, nt.21] We will look now at some of the principles of food preparation that may bolster mineral intake.

"Meaty" Vegetable Dishes: The Secrets of Seasoning

Although meat is not an ideal source of trace minerals, it is certainly ample compared with the processed vegetable foods such as white bread, sweetened desserts, and french fried potatoes that usually accompany it. Part of the appeal of meat is probably its ability to satisfy one's need for the minerals that are absent from the rest of the meat-eater's diet. In fact, besides its protein content, it may be the abundance of minerals that prompts us to describe a food as "meaty." If one is to successfully eliminate meat and not suffer a craving for it or a deficiency of trace minerals, then one must find another way of supplying them.

One important source of minerals such as calcium and manganese is fresh, cooked, green—preferably leafy—vegetables. The assortment of vegetables used, the way in which they are prepared, and the way in which they are grown are all important in determining the quantity and variety of trace minerals they bring. Most people do not have access to organically grown produce in any quantity, and may have no way of finding out any details about the way in which the vegetables they have purchased were grown. Therefore the selection of an appropriate variety of vegetable foods and the techniques used for preparing them come to be of prime importance in preparing a vegetable dish that is a concentrated source of minerals and that will, as a result, be appealing and "meaty."

Seasonings may be one of our ways of adding minerals that are missing to our food. Classical Indian vegetarian cooking, for example, relies heavily on the use of herbs and spices. Although herbs and spices are generally used in relatively small quantities, they have been found to contain enormous concentrations of trace minerals.[135] Thyme, for example, contains 100 times as much chromium as does meat, and 400 times as much manganese. Black pepper, cloves, ginger, and bay leaves have also been tested and found to be extraordinarily rich in trace elements. It has been suggested that their intensity of taste might be due to their concentration of such minerals.[135]

This may explain why combining spices and seasonings skillfully is given so much attention in classical traditions of vegetarian cooking. Their purpose may be much more than the mere creation of taste sensations that can replace the flavor of meat. It's possible that instead they provide from a different source what was nutritionally essential and appealing in the meat.

Flavor Bases: The Horizons Beyond Meat

In most meat-based meals it is the meat that is used to provide a flavor base. Even in basically meatless foods the flavor base used is often meat. The vegetarian who orders what appears to be a simple vegetable soup may well discover, much to his chagrin, that it is made with meat stock. Meat stock is used because vegetables are considered bland. The vast majority of ordinary recipes, even those for grains, beans, and vegetables, have meat or some meat product such as bacon bits or chicken broth to give flavor.

Vegetarian food must derive its flavor base some other way. The Japanese and Chinese often use fermented soy products, such as miso or tamari, for this purpose, because they have a strong taste that resembles meat to some extent. Because of unresolved questions about the toxic effects of many molds, and the undesirable tamasic aspects of fermented foods in general, such condiments are probably best used sparingly and infrequently.

But another way of providing a basic flavor is through the use of spices. This is the classical Indian vegetarian approach, and in its most healthful form it relies on turmeric, cumin, and coriander as a foundation for most seasoning. There are a number of reasons for choosing them, some of which have to do with their medicinal effects. But what's most interesting about them from a culinary point of view is that if they are well browned without burning they provide a rich but relatively neutral flavor base, very much like beef stock or soy sauce. Lighter browning will create a different effect, more suitable for the dishes usually seasoned with chicken stock. If onions are added to the roasted spices and also browned, their taste is further enriched and intensified. This seasoning mixture supplies a satisfying basic flavor for beans or vegetables that not only replaces meat but provides more interest and more possibilities for variety.

The choice of basic spices or their proportions can be modified on occasion, or other spices, such as ginger, cloves, cardamom, black pepper, or mustard seed, can be used to complement them, as can other seasoning vegetables besides onions, such as garlic, green peppers, mushrooms, celery, tomatoes, and so on. These modifications will transform the basic flavor to such an extent that it seems different and doesn't become boring or repetitious.

According to the Ayurvedic perspective, such seasonings also have a medicinal effect that promotes digestion and helps reduce the tendency to cause gas. This makes them particularly useful in

Whole Mung Beans

1 cup dried whole mung

1 large onion, chopped

1 medium green pepper,
chopped

1 cup mushrooms, chopped

1 large tomato, scalded, peeled,
and mashed or pureed

3 T clarified butter

½ tsp turmeric

1 tsp ground cumin

1½ tsp ground coriander

½ tsp black mustard seed
(optional)

1 tsp salt

Pick and wash beans; soak overnight. Cover with water, plus an inch or two, and cook in a three-quart pot until tender, adding boiling water as necessary. In a large iron skillet fry butterfat until well browned, then add mustard seed. When they begin to pop, add onion. Fry until golden brown. Then add green pepper and mushrooms and fry until onions are dark brown. Add tomato and fry briefly. Pour some of cooked beans into skillet and stir, then put everything into bean pot. Add salt and enough boiling water to cook another 5-10 minutes. Serve with rice, a cooked green vegetable, and flatbread.

Source: Ballentine, *Himalayan Mountain Cookery.*[107]

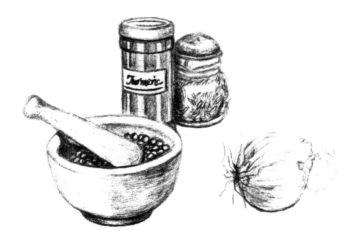

the preparation of bean dishes. Some of them, unfortunately, have side effects that are undesirable, such as the irritation of the intestinal tract that results from very hot spices like chili peppers. For this reason they are best used only in small quantities and intermittently. Turmeric, cumin, and coriander, however, are mild and beneficial, and can be regularly used in a vegetarian regimen without difficulty.

Vegetable dishes, when properly prepared, well cooked (though not overcooked), and seasoned with the appropriate herbs and spices, can be very satisfying and rich in the same nutrients that meat provides, without the risks to health that meat and poultry entail.

By the end of Phase 2, one should have not only eliminated red meat and poultry, but also made some additional changes that will result in a diet that is far superior to what is current today.

Goals for Phase 2

1. To have eliminated:
- red meat
- refined sugars
- **fowl**
- **refined flour**

2. To have added:
- a grain/legume combination **twice a week**
- a fresh, cooked, leafy green vegetable at least **twice a week**

3. To take regularly:
- **two pieces** of fresh fruit **each day**
- a green salad **once a day**
- a fresh, cooked, green or yellow vegetable **each day**
- at least **one serving** of whole grains **a day**

PHASE 3

FISH

By the time one reaches the point of taking a critical look at fish, not only will meat and poultry have been eliminated from the diet, but other constructive changes will have been made, too. These include the elimination of high-sugar and high-phosphate foods and beverages, packaged salty and sweet snack foods, excessively oily and greasy foods, and most foods made with refined flours and sweeteners. A daily ration of two or three pieces of fresh fruit, a generous amount of fresh, cooked, green vegetables, and several servings of whole grains taken in combination with a cooked legume should have become a regular routine. After a few months such shifts in diet will ordinarily yield a considerable increase in energy and vitality. A greater sense of well-being is often experienced by those who have established these new habits. At this point many persons feel quite comfortable and are content to continue with the Phase 2 diet for some time.

Certainly that's a reasonable course to follow. Coastal populations and inland fishing peoples are often found among the groups known for their good health and longevity. Diseases like atherosclerosis, which are so prevalent in meat-eaters, are almost unknown in areas where only fish and plant foods are consumed. Weston Price, a dentist who did pioneering work on nutrition and anthropology in the 1920s, traveled around the world to study primitive peoples in their native settings following their established diets. He commented: "During these investigations . . . I have been impressed with the superior quality of the human stock developed by nature whenever a liberal source of seafoods exists."[1]

More than 70% of the earth's surface is covered with water. This provides a vast source of food for humans. If fish are taken judiciously from lakes and oceans, the protein needs of huge populations can be met without upsetting the ecological balance of the biosphere. In fact, in some cases, the appropriate harvesting of fish can help maintain that balance.

It is perhaps for all these reasons that seafood is increasingly being recognized as providing a sensible alternative to meat. The consumption of fresh and frozen seafood rose by 42% between 1960 and 1976.[2] In the last few years it has increased even more rapidly—spurred on by a widening recognition of the problems with meat and poultry.

Lean fish, such as flounder, haddock, whiting, and cod, contain as little as 1% fat and have a reputation, considered well merited by nutritionists, of being light and easily digested.[3] Fish protein is equal in value to that of meat or poultry. Unlike most red meat and poultry, which comes from domesticated animals, fish is generally caught from the wild. For this reason it is less given to the diseases and disorders that result from overcrowding and artificial environments. Moreover, fish are cold-blooded aquatic animals and thus less likely than warm-blooded cattle and birds to harbor the microbes that create human disease. Finfish are generally quite safe in this respect, though shellfish can carry disease-causing agents if gathered from polluted waters.

Marine fish are a rich source of trace minerals such as selenium and iodine that may be deficient in land plants and animals. Because humans descended from animals that evolved in the sea, our biochemistry is based on a mineral balance very similar to that of seawater, and the wealth of trace elements in seawater will be found in dependable quantities and proper proportions in seafoods. Small fish such as sardines and anchovies that are eaten whole along with their bones may even be a useful source of calcium.

Fish also provide a reliable ration of vitamin B_{12}, a nutrient that is not present in plant foods and whose lack could become a serious problem for those who have eliminated meat and poultry. The oils of fish are rich in the fat-soluble vitamins A and D. They also have other advantages that are just now beginning to be identified. In order to understand the action of fish oils and their place in the diet, we will look more closely at their composition and their relation to the essential fatty acids.

FISH OILS AND THE ESSENTIAL FATTY ACIDS

The effects of fish oil on blood cholesterol have created quite a stir recently. Both the popular press and the scientific journals have carried numerous articles acclaiming the virtues of one of the constituents of fish oil, known as eicosapentaenoic acid, mercifully abbreviated EPA. Diets high in this component of fish oil seem to protect against coronary heart disease.[4-8]

It has been known for some time that Greenland Eskimos consuming their customary diet rich in fish oils show a strikingly lower incidence of heart disease than comparable groups in Denmark.[4] Japanese on a traditional diet that includes substantial amounts of seafood also have unusually little heart disease.[5]

Though heart attacks are less common in Japan in general than they are in Europe or North America, there are differences between different groups within Japan, too. It looks as though these differences may be due, at least in part, to the quantity of fish consumed. When the fishing peoples of a small coastal village in Japan were compared with farmers from an inland community, there were marked differences. It was found that the fishermen and their wives, whose fish consumption was nearly three times that of the farmers, had almost twice as much EPA in their blood and a significantly lower incidence of both heart attacks and strokes.[5]

Since populations in the Far East are often tradition-bound and very stable, one might conclude that the different genetic makeup of the two Japanese communities was responsible. But a recent study in Sweden showed a clear-cut relationship between the amount of fish eaten and mortality from coronary heart disease, even when the pairs of persons being compared were twins, and even after adjustments were made for such differences as smoking habits, obesity, and blood pressure.[8] The higher the fish intake, the lower the death rate from heart attacks.

Recent research suggests that EPA protects against heart attacks primarily by decreasing the blood's tendency to clot. Heart attacks occur when the small arteries supplying blood to the wall of the heart become obstructed. This obstruction is due partly to cholesterol deposits, but will also often be aggravated by the thickening and partial clotting or sludging of the blood in those small arteries already narrowed by atherosclerosis. In fact, for some reason, people who develop atherosclerosis have an exaggerated tendency for their blood cells to get sticky and for their blood to sludge and clot easily. EPA interferes with the clotting mechanisms, slowing coagulation. Moreover, it also seems to decrease blood levels of triglycerides and cholesterol, which should help prevent an earlier phase of the disease, the formation of the fatty deposits along the arterial walls.[9, nt.1]

While fish oils, because of their EPA, may act to lower blood levels of cholesterol, seafood may contain some cholesterol itself, though probably not enough to have a major effect. At one time it was thought that shellfish such as lobster and shrimp were especially high in cholesterol, but subsequent refinements in laboratory technique have shown that part of what had been measured were substances similar enough to cholesterol to show up as positive on the test but different enough to be metabolized along separate pathways and thus incapable of increasing the risk of arterial disease.

In fact, when patients with high blood cholesterol levels and high triglyceride levels ate mackerel (a moderate- to high-fat fish) for a period and then switched to herring (a fish with almost no fat or oil), it was noted that their levels of high-density lipoproteins (HDL), the faction of fatty substance in the blood that has a protective effect against heart disease, were higher on the oilier mackerel diet.[11, 13] Though the percentage of EPA in the oils of different types of fish varies, the variation is not so great, according to experts in Finland. They contend that

Fish by Fat Content

Low-fat 0-2%	Medium-fat 2-7%	High-fat 8-15%
cod	halibut	herring
haddock	Pacific mackerel	eel
whiting	mullet	Atlantic mackerel
flounder	trout	whitefish
pike	sardine	shad

Source: Nettleton: *Seafood Nutrition.*[14]

when attempting to choose a variety of fish that would be most beneficial, the total amount of oil is the important consideration, and advise that the fatter the fish, the more beneficial its dietary effect.[15] Since the risk for cardiovascular disease is also higher in persons with hypertension, it is relevant here that in both animal studies[16] and human patients[11,17] fish or fish oil have been found to produce mild but significant decreases in blood pressure.

Extracted EPA is now being marketed in concentrated form for those who don't want to eat fish but want the benefits of fish oil. There is even a recent report of the successful use of EPA to treat migraine headaches, suggesting that it may also reduce vascular spasm—another effect that could contribute to preventing the occlusion of coronary arteries.[18]

Thus, EPA may act in a variety of ways to protect against heart attacks: (1) decreasing the stickiness of the blood, (2) improving the lipid profile (lowering total blood cholesterol and triglycerides and raising HDL), (3) lowering blood pressure, and (4) possibly preventing spasm in the arteries.

EPA Supplements

Enthusiasm for the benefits of EPA has led to cases of overzealous dosing with the purified fatty acid. Fish oils, like other fats and oils, occur in nature mostly in the form of triglycerides. These molecules are made up of three fat chains joined by a glycerol (see diagram). The fat chains are called fatty acids, since the end that attaches has an acidic structure that enables it to react with and lock into the glycerol molecule that holds the three chains together. Each triglyceride found in the diet, such as a molecule of fish oil, will be made up of an assorted selection of three fatty acids. When these chains are split off, one can make a pure, concentrated preparation of a single fatty acid. Commercially available EPA is a very concentrated source of the active fatty acid, being about 75% pure.[19]

With such a preparation, taking six capsules three times a day would have approximately the same effect as 1¼ pounds of moderately oily fish. While that's not a huge amount, it's more than most people take in on a regular basis. Japanese fishermen took only an average of ½ pound a day. Patients anxious to protect themselves against heart diseases who have swallowed a dozen capsules a day have found themselves bleeding and have had difficulty stopping it.[nt.2]

Numerous observers have reported that Greenland Eskimos, the same population that has a very low incidence of heart disease, is also given to frequent episodes of bleeding. Several Arctic explorers commented on the frequent nosebleeds suffered by the natives. One of them noticed that he, himself, also began to have the problem when he failed to bring along his own rations and found it necessary to follow the Eskimos' diet. The tendency in these Eskimos to cough up blood and to have blood in the urine

The Triglyceride Molecule

were also reported, as well as hemorrhages after childbirth that were difficult to control and that were associated with maternal mortality. One physician in 1911 wrote: "The Eskimos are strongly inclined to bleeding. The tendency almost amounts to hemophilia."[20]

This would suggest that a moderate amount of fish in the diet, maybe ¼ pound a day on the average, might be a useful adjunct to other dietary changes in preventing heart disease.[nt.3] But it seems unwise to use pure fish oil or EPA as a medicinal agent in an attempt to control a tendency to arterial disease that is all the while being aggravated by a fatty, low-fiber diet.

The Essential Fatty Acids

EPA can also be produced in the body from linolenic acid, one of the essential fatty acids. Essential fatty acids are those fat chains human cells cannot readily synthesize but that are needed for proper functioning. Customarily three of them are mentioned: linoleic, linolenic, and arachidonic.

They are all polyunsaturated fatty acids. That is, there are some empty spots or double bonds in the carbon chains that constitute their basic structure (see figure below). These double

Saturated and Unsaturated Fatty Acids

Saturated

Monounsaturated

Polyunsaturated

*acid end attaches to glyceral

bonds lower the melting point; the more unsaturated spots, the more liquid is the fat. Polyunsaturates such as corn oil or soy oil remain liquid even under refrigeration, while mono-unsaturates such as olive oil begin to solidify. Fats such as butter or lard, which contain a higher percentage of saturated fatty acids (such as stearic acid), will remain semi-solid even at room temperature.

Linoleic acid is one of the most common fatty acids in vegetable oils. In a diet in which vegetable oils are not used for cooking and in which unrefined plant foods that have their own oil content are seldom eaten, one might end up short of linoleic acid. Meat and potatoes, for example, with white bread, cheese and eggs, and with lard as a cooking medium but with scanty vegetables, could produce a genuine deficiency of linoleic acid.

The likelihood of such a deficiency developing is increased by the fact that a high intake of saturated animal fats is thought to increase one's need for the essential fatty acids. Cases of eczema emerging in children in such diets decades ago were dramatically relieved by doses of supplementary vegetable oil, and earned polyunsaturates a reputation among practical-minded nutritionists for curing eczema.

Though a generation of hapless children have choked down tablespoons of oil, little good has come of it, since a dietary deficiency of linoleic acid is nearly impossible these days. Everyone gets lots of linoleic-rich vegetable oil now, even meat-eaters, because such oils are used for deep frying, for salad dressings, and in many prepared foods. Moreover, when it was found that polyunsaturated vegetable oils could lower blood cholesterol levels, their use was widely encouraged. In fact, Americans presently get about 10% of their calories from the linoleic acid of such oils—an amount much higher than necessary to meet essential fatty acid requirements.

The primary use of the essential fatty acids is as raw materials from which are produced certain critical hormone-like substances that control cellular metabolism. These substances go by such names as prostaglandins, prostacyclins, and thromboxanes. They are among the most potent of all biological agents, producing dramatic effects in only minute doses.

water-soluble part

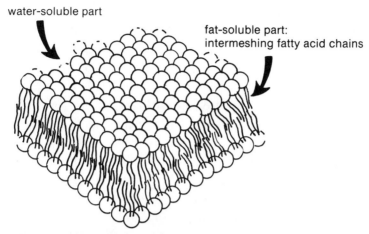

fat-soluble part:
intermeshing fatty acid chains

Structure of the Lipid Bilayer Membrane

Source: Mead: *Free Radical Mechanisms.*[21]

Much of their activity revolves around the cell membrane, an important crossroads and a critical obstacle that all nutrients must traverse if they are to reach the inside of the cell. Not only do prostaglandins and related substances frequently serve to facilitate or block movement of other molecules through the membrane, they are often manufactured from components of the membrane itself. The membrane, an ingenious layering of fatty acids and phosphates-containing proteins, includes a center layer made up of a mixture of fatty acids (see figure above), some of which are precisely the ones used to make prostaglandins. Manufacturing them on site, where they can do their work and then be broken down quickly, allows their potent effects to be controlled.

It is thought that EPA slows clotting by becoming incorporated into the membrane structure of blood cells[nt.4] and replacing arachidonic acid, one of the three essential fatty acids. If the membranes contain mostly arachidonic acid, then clotting is promoted. If most of this is replaced by EPA, then it's not.

Omega-3 and Omega-6

Until recently, everything written in nutrition books about essential fatty acids emphasized linoleic acid, the predominant fatty acid in common vegetable oils such as safflower oil and corn oil. Linoleic acid is readily converted in the body to arachidonic acid, the membrane constituent that is used to make clot-promoting thromboxanes. These two make up part of a sequence of fat chains produced one from the other, each of which has its first double bond at a position six carbons from the end. For this reason they are called "omega-6" fatty acids.

Now researchers concerned about accelerated clotting and its role in heart disease and strokes are talking about the ratio of EPA to arachidonic acid. EPA is part of a different series. It is made not from linoleic acid but from linolenic acid. (The spelling of the two fatty acids is similar, but their metabolic roles are very different.) The fatty acids of this series have the double bonds further toward the end, and are called "omega-3." (See figure on p. 153.)

Fish oils have a high content of omega-3 fatty acids; most of the commonly used vegetable oils are predominantly omega-6. It's increasingly thought that too much of the omega-6 variety and too little of the omega-3 can increase clotting and precipitate heart attacks and strokes, as well as aggravating a variety of other disorders such as allergic tendencies.[22] At any rate, proportion may be more important in the case of the essential fatty acids—and other oils in the diet—than actual quantity. Drastic increases in any one, whether it's one of the omega-3s from extra fish oil or omega-6s from added vegetable oil, is likely to be unwise. A balance is best, and will generally follow from a diet of mostly plant foods that contain adequate quantities of both linoleic and linolenic acids.

Moreover, trying to solve problems by taking supplementary doses of oils of any kind brings a new set of problems, since oils are peculiarly susceptible to deterioration. Their double bonds make neighboring hydrogen atoms unstable, and oxygen easily combines with them. The oxidation of unsaturated fatty acids destroys their flavor and gives them an off odor. They are then said to be rancid.

Bottles of vegetable oils, especially those with multiple double bonds, the polyunsaturated oils, and nuts and seeds that contain large amounts of such oils readily go rancid when exposed to air.

EPA and Essential Fatty Acids

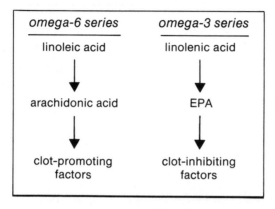

Fish oils will do the same; rancid fish oils are responsible for much of the objectionable fish odor of seafood that is not fresh. Fish just caught and immediately cooked is a different matter altogether, and its appeal is responsible for much of the enthusiasm of week-end fishermen. But most of the fish consumed today is not of that sort.

PROBLEMS WITH FISH: SANITATION, PCBs, AND MERCURY

A majority of the fish that is commercially available is caught at sea by large fishing boats. Because the fishing vessels stay out for days or weeks before filling their holds and returning to port, and because fishery products are among the most perishable of foodstuffs, maintaining the catch in good condition is a challenge of considerable proportions. Storage conditions must be carefully controlled to slow the growth of microorganisms and minimize spoilage. The rapidity with which deterioration occurs will depend on a number of factors.

Fish caught on a line, or caught from near the surface of deeper waters, will have lower initial bacterial counts than those that are trawled by dragging a net along the bottom. The trawl net is pulled through the sediment, which has the highest counts of microbes. How the fish are handled after they are brought to the surface can increase contamination extensively. Since fish do not have a sphincter muscle at the anal opening, any pressure applied will cause the intestinal contents to be squeezed out and to spill over the rest of the catch. Pressure is exerted when the net is hauled aboard, when the fish are piled on the deck, and during storage in ice.

Shrimp fishing presents typical problems. After one to three hours of dragging the trawl net along the bottom, it is hauled on board and emptied. Contamination from the bottom sediment results in a bacterial count at this point that ranges up to over a million per gram.[23] To put this figure in perspective, salmonella counts as low as 1 to 10 organisms per gram have caused infection in humans.[24] Although salmonella is not one of the predominant organisms found in raw shrimp, since it does not grow well in the intestinal tract of fish, nonetheless bottom-feeding fish and shellfish are prone to contamination with it when they come from coastal waters that have suffered some pollution by sewage.[25]

The shrimp trawler will remain offshore for 4 to 20 days. Properly packed in ice, the temperature of the shrimp can be maintained at near freezing so that it will remain in excellent condition for a day or two. After that, the number of bacteria begins to increase rapidly.[23] The shrimp toward the bottom of the hold have a higher bacterial count, due to the melting ice that carries microbes down from the upper layers. The weight of the shrimp and the ice atop them will also tend to crush those at the bottom. This damage, plus the bacteria washed down from above, further increases the rate of deterioration. As with other fish, under these circumstances there is also a certain degree of leaching of nutrients by the ice water.

By the time they reach port, most fish have already suffered considerable contamination, damage, and microbial growth. They usually proceed from port to a processing plant, where they are put up for distribution. As we have seen with meat and poultry, the processing steps through which the fish must go, such as gutting and filleting, tend to spread organisms from the surface slime layer into the final product, further encouraging spoilage.

After dressing, the fish may be canned, pickled or even dried, but nowadays most are frozen. Though canned fish has been largely abandoned by today's consumer in favor of frozen fish, there remains one conspicuous exception: tuna. In fact, the consumption of canned tuna has increased dramatically in recent years and now accounts for more than a quarter of all fish consumed by Americans.[2]

Riding on the wave of the current enthusiasm for fish as a healthier alternative to meat, "the chicken of the sea" has established a firm place for itself in American kitchens. It's compact, simple, and quick to use. It's not so "fishy" as many fishes, and everyone's favorite shortcut cookbook has temptingly easy recipes for tuna casserole dinners and tasty tunafish salads. But does the tuna can really capture the health-giving benefits of the fresh item? Probably not. Assays indicate, for example, that fresh tuna has more than twice as much vitamin B_6 as canned tuna, and over 50% more pantothenic acid, another important B vitamin.[26]

Frozen fish generally retains a higher percentage of vitamins, though there may be some losses. Losses will increase if fish are allowed to thaw out after freezing. Even when care is taken, fish will frequently thaw as they are transferred from processing plant to wholesaler and from wholesale warehouse to the retail market. This thawing and refreezing takes its toll on the quality of the food. At each thawing, a certain amount of fluid, or "drip," which is rich in nutrients, is lost from the fish.[26] With refreezing, reactions catalyzed by enzymes are accelerated. It is thought that freezing and thawing disrupt the subcellular compartments that contain these enzymes, releasing them and allowing them to act on nutritionally important cellular components. The result is vitamin destruction, protein loss, and acceleration of the rancidification of oils.

Although texture and taste of the fish suffer accordingly each time the process is repeated, refreezing even once has adverse effects on the nutritional value of fish. In one study, loss of lysine was 31% in a refrozen lot, while it was only 9% in fish that had been frozen fresh.[26] This is a substantial difference, and quite an important one for the person who is largely vegetarian but uses fish as a supplementary protein, since lysine, as mentioned in the previous chapter, is a common limiting amino acid in meals based on grains.

Fish Inspection

Standards for the processing and handling of seafoods are not mandatory. This is quite different from the controls for meat and poultry. The USDA inspects meat and requires it to comply with standards set by the agency. The surveillance of fishery products has evolved in a different direction, and may actually, as a result, be more effective.

The Commerce Department provides inspection of fish processing plants at their request, and they pay the cost. They are motivated by a desire to market their products to large institutions and retail chains. These big buyers don't want the liability of suits from customers who have fallen ill from tainted fish, so they may refuse to buy from processors who aren't certified by the National Seafood Quality and Inspection Laboratory.

The result is that there has been an increasing eagerness on the part of processors to be inspected. Currently nearly 60% of frozen fish on the market has been voluntarily inspected through this process. Since the plants themselves foot the bill, the Seafood Inspection Program is immune to government budget crunches. Whereas meat inspectors sometimes become relatively ineffectual circuit riders, showing up at plants with decreasing frequency as funds dwindle, seafood inspectors can afford to remain on site. Moreover, they are rotated every 6 to 8 months, thus preventing the development of the undue influence that can be a complication of long-term involvement.

A separate agency was created to handle shellfish surveillance after a major outbreak of typhoid fever was traced to sewage-polluted oysters in 1925. Shellfish present certain unique problems since they are bivalves or filter-feeders. That means they pump water through their bodies, filtering out its contents for their food. The volume of water pumped by a single oyster can amount to 2½ gallons in an hour. As a result, shellfish have an extraordinary capacity to concentrate the microorganisms found in the water. They carry a resident population of bacteria that runs upwards of a million per gram of tissue.

Oysters and mussels harvested for human use are usually grown in estuarine areas that receive some waste from land sources. By feeding in polluted waters they concentrate the contaminating microbes such as salmonella and the viruses that cause hepatitis. Though certain waters have been approved, bootleg fishermen abound, and "large quantities of shellfish harvested from uncontrolled areas still enter the human food supply and represent a considerable hazard."[27]

When shellfish were obtained from five collecting stations, 7% to 20% were found to be contaminated with salmonella. Another survey found that 40% of the mussels tested harbored these bacteria.[28] Bottom-feeders such as catfish and crayfish are also, like shellfish, especially likely to be carriers of salmonella.

One method of dealing with the possible contamination of filter-feeders is to put them, after harvest but while they are still alive, into clean water and allow their natural pumping mechanisms to flush out the contaminants. After 24 to 48 hours of this they are usually considered safe.[29] Though no cases of infectious hepatitis have been reported from flushed shellfish, it is not clear how effective the procedure is for viruses. Experimental infection of oysters with polio virus and subsequent flushing left residual levels of the virus that were enough to cause disease.[30]

In addition, experimentally contaminated oysters were found to retain salmonella for at least 49 days.[31] This suggests that flushing is not a foolproof measure and that clean beds are needed for the production and harvesting of shellfish. Yet an international commission on the subject has stated: "The spread of human habitation and activity in the inshore marine and estuarine waters all over the world makes it increasingly unlikely that purity (particularly freedom from virus contamination) can be maintained in all growing areas."[32]

The greatest danger of illness from shellfish is incurred when they are eaten raw. Clams or oysters on the half shell are particularly risky, and are a common cause of hepatitis. Cooking makes them safer but may not be completely reliable; a bacterial count of over a million per gram has been found in crabs that were boiled for 30 minutes.[33] It is difficult for normal cooking to rid such seafoods of microbes if they were caught in waters that were heavily polluted. Though it may be getting worse, the problem is hardly new. Pollution of populated coastal areas with sewage dates back to early times. It is perhaps for this reason that Judaic dietary law forbade the use of seafoods such as crabs.

PCBs and Other Toxins

Of course, water can carry other pollutants besides sewage and its disease-causing microbes. Pollution with toxic chemicals and metals such as the mercury and cadmium found in industrial wastes are currently a major concern. PCBs (polychlorinated biphenyls) have been the cause of much public attention since they are toxic in minute doses, quite persistent in the environment, and tend to accumulate in food chains, as was pointed out earlier.

Though PCBs can be found in soils and groundwater, coastal seawater and lakes and rivers near industrial sites show the highest levels. This is especially true of bottom sediments, which may contain extremely high concentrations. Fish caught in the Great Lakes have been found to have the highest levels in the U.S. Though manufacture of PCBs has been curtailed and rigorous standards set for their use and handling, the persistence of the chemical in fish remains troublesome.[34] The Michigan Department of Natural Resources issued an advisory in 1977 warning fishermen to eat no more than ½ pound per week of contaminated Great Lakes fish, and suggesting that women of childbearing age avoid altogether those types of fish that had been found to have high levels of PCBs. Like many other toxic chemicals that are deposited in waters and find their way into fish, PCBs are fat-soluble, and are most concentrated in the fatty part of the fish. Therefore, high-fat fish have the highest levels.

A study in Sweden found that the milk of nursing mothers who regularly ate fatty fish from the Baltic Sea had higher levels of PCBs and pesticide residues than that of mothers who ate a regular meat-based diet. The lowest levels of contaminants were found in the breastmilk of lactovegetarians.[35] To minimize the risks that come from chemicals in the fish oil, health officials recommended trimming away the skin with as much fat as possible, and broiling the fish so that a major part of the fat is rendered out.

This poses something of a dilemma for the health-conscious fish-eater, who is told on the one hand to take the fattiest fish he can find in order to get more omega-3 fatty acids, such as EPA, but warned, on the other hand, to avoid high-fat fish because of its content of such toxins as PCBs. One can, of course, choose one's fish carefully, taking high-fat fish from deep ocean waters and low-fat (if any) fish from areas like the Great Lakes. But the simplest solution may lie in a different direction.

It has been recently discovered that certain plant foods are quite rich in omega-3 oils. These include walnuts, legumes, tofu, and seaweed.[36] It has long been known that beans and peas have a protective effect against heart disease (see pp. 52-53, 97). Perhaps their content of omega-3 fatty acids is part of the reason why. One green vegetable, used extensively by the peoples of the Mediterranean area, where the incidence of both heart disease and cancer is low, is an especially good source of omega-3 oils. Known as purslane in North America and England, where it is considered a weed, it is richer in omega-3 fatty acids than any other plant so far examined.[37]

Of course plant foods are quite low in PCBs and the chlorinated hydrocarbon pesticides, and they generally bring along ample fiber that may help carry out of the body what does get in. Plant foods are also low in toxic heavy metals such as mercury, which can contaminate seafoods. Mercury is another subject that demands the attention of the fish-eater. Mercury levels in fish have aroused a good deal of anxiety—more, some experts feel, than is really merited.

Mercury in Fish

In 1953, several Japanese men who fished the waters of Minamata Bay, and the members of their families, began to develop a strange neurological disease. Their limbs became weak, their vision dimmed, and they lost their ability to coordinate their movements. Many of those affected became progressively weaker and gradually paralyzed. Some lapsed into comas and died. Though over the following years more and more people in the area succumbed and autopsies on them showed deterioration of the brain, the cause remained a mystery. As household cats and seabirds fell ill with similar disorders, investigators began to suspect fish as a source of the disease. After six years, 111 cases had been reported, 41 of which were fatal.

It was only in 1968, 15 years later, that a full report was published, showing agreement on the origin of the illness: it was mercury poisoning from contaminated fish. The waters of Minamata Bay were polluted with water from a chemical plant where mercury was used as a manufacturing catalyst. Meanwhile, in 1962, another outbreak had occurred among 26 people (with 5 deaths) along the Agano River in Niigata, Japan. This was also due to contaminated fish from a chemical plant. Additional incidents have occurred in Iraq, Pakistan, and Guatemala, where farmers had eaten mercury-treated grain intended for planting.

At about the same time, scientists from Sweden reported that a survey of fish caught there revealed high mercury levels, while other scientists who checked the feathers of birds in museums found that mercury levels had increased markedly after 1940.[38] Lethal levels of mercury were discovered in animals found dead in the Swedish countryside.[39] At that point the Swedish government banned fish with mercury levels above a one part per million (1 ppm) limit.

By 1970 contaminated fish were identified on the Great Lakes, and the FDA seized shipments of fish that were considered dangerous. There was widespread alarm: Should fish be considered unfit for use? Concern about the safety of swordfish, for example, virtually ended the industry.

As is often the case, the danger was initially exaggerated. Careful research showed the problem to be much less grave than was at first thought. The truth is, mercury has been widespread throughout nature as far back as we can know. The earth's crust contains approximately 1 ppm, as do groundwater samples, though seawater contains only a fraction of that. Metallic mercury is heavy and tends to settle out of the water, so it is more concentrated on the floor of the ocean. Most of that comes from erosion of soil; humanity's pollution of the environment constitutes only a minor contribution. Moreover, this heavy mercury on the depths of the ocean floor seems relatively inactive, as deepwater fish actually show lower levels of mercury than those from shallow waters.

Nor have fish been becoming more polluted—actually, the bones of prehistoric fish show more mercury than those currently being caught,[40] and museum specimens of tuna caught around the turn of the century have almost 50% more mercury than those caught today. What has changed is that modern industry has produced a few small but concentratred pockets of mercury waste that can cause toxic levels in fish, such as those in Japan. These are isolated incidents and their severity is dependent on the presence of a specific compound, methyl mercury.

Methyl Mercury Versus Elemental Mercury

The vast majority of mercury in the environmental water and food supply exists as elemental mercury, the silver liquid one sees in a clinical thermometer. It's a heavy metallic substance that has intrigued the curious since ancient times since it is the only metal that remains liquid at room temperature. This quicksilver, though reputed to be toxic, is only mildly so. One expert on mercury claims that swallowing up to a pound of it will produce no significant ill effects.[41] From this perspective, the distribution of mercury through soils, waterways, and plant and animal life is natural and innocuous. As one prominent authority on heavy metal pollution said: "The whole mercury scare could be a gigantic scientific misconception, inadvertent, to be sure, but still false."[40]

A similar complacency is not appropriate, however, when one turns to certain mercury compounds such as methyl mercury. This highly dangerous substance is estimated to be 50 times as toxic as mercury itself, and stays in the fat and in the nervous system 14 times as long.[40] Moreover, it is quite well absorbed from the digestive tract,[42] whereas only a minute fraction of elemental mercury is absorbed. It is methyl mercury that is used to coat seeds so that they won't mold, and it was methyl mercury that was present in the waters of Minamata Bay.

Methyl mercury more easily crosses the placental and blood/ brain barriers. Thus, children born retarded or with cerebral palsy have been found among mothers poisoned with methyl mercury,[42] and in adults it can produce a picture of irritability, fatigue, depression, and loss of memory. "As mad as a hatter" was a phrase used to describe the absentminded and short-tempered felt hat processers who used a similar though less toxic mercury compound in their work. Mercury poisoning can also result in tremors that resemble Parkinson's disease. In fact, Swedish investigators have found evidence of mercury exposure in a high percentage of patients with Parkinson's disease and have raised the question of a causal connection.[43, nt.5] Unfortunately, while methyl mercury is accumulating in the nervous system, there may be no recognizable symptoms for many years.[44]

Happily, in foods of plant origin, little or none of the mercury present is normally in the form of methyl mercury. In meat and dairy products the low levels of mercury present can include a small proportion of the methyl compound, presumably from residues in feeds containing fish meal or treated grains. Unfortunately, opinions differ remarkably when it comes to how much of the mercury in fish is in the form of methyl mercury and how much is in the metallic elemental form. Some experts say that most of the mercury in fish is present as highly toxic methyl mercury compounds.[42] Others vehemently disagree.[40]

Though the issue remains controversial, we do know that mercury is converted to the methyl form by certain microorganisms in the water. Algae in some areas have been found to contain high concentrations of methyl mercury. This may result in substantial methyl mercury levels in fish that have fed on them. It would, in addition, suggest that seaweed and algae preparations intended for human consumption (such as spirulina) should be monitored for methyl mercury.

Biological methylation has also been demonstrated in the soil and in the intestinal tract, and such a transformation can also take place in the mouth, as well. The bacteria that cause dental plaque have been demonstrated to convert mercury to its methyl form.[45] They have a ready source of metallic mercury: the silver-tin-mercury amalgam used in dental fillings. This mercury is not only readily available for methylation, it can also be directly absorbed as mercury vapor.

One of the well-known toxic effects of mercury is to make the gums spongy and unhealthy. It is possible that the widespread use of silver-mercury fillings has contributed to the nearly universal incidence of gum disease in America, setting up a situation in which the constant overgrowth of bacteria in unhealthy gums can provide the conditions for the methylation of mercury and the perpetuation of a vicious cycle.

Symptom pictures that bear more than a superficial resemblance to mercury toxicity are being reported with increasing frequency by physicians as well as dentists. Many of these patients are found to have a diet high in fish. It may be that although neither the fish nor the silver-mercury amalgam alone is sufficient to cause problems, the combination of the two is enough to do so. If fish consumption is high, it may be sufficient to cause toxicity all alone. Indians in northern Canada who eat over a pound of fish a day through much of the year are showing signs of mercury poisoning such as partial blindness. Fish in the area are highly contaminated.[46, nt.6]

Just why such cases of mercury toxicity are increasing is not completely clear. It may be that we are just recognizing it more frequently. It seems more likely, however, that it is the result of a combination of factors: a heavy load of toxic substances in the body, a deficiency of protective nutrients, and perhaps a disturbance of the delicate balances of the ecological systems that regulate the rate and frequency of conversion of the less harmful forms of mercury to those that are more dangerous. It has been suggested that wastes dumped into the waters may supply compounds that encourage the growth of microorganisms that convert mercury to its methyl form.[41]

Though the gravity of the threat of mercury toxicity remains controversial, even most skeptics seem to think it reasonable to avoid fish like swordfish that are caught at a more advanced age and have had longer to accumulate mercury, and thus show the highest levels. Fish of all sorts taken from waters where there is intensive industrialization are particularly likely to be unsafe. A recent study in West Germany of 136 persons who regularly consumed fish from the River Elbe found a correlation between the amount of fish eaten and blood levels of both mercury and pesticide residues.[47]

Natural Toxins in Fish

Not all toxins in seafood are man-made, the result of pollution, or a consequence of man's disturbance of ecological balances. Some fish toxins have been around since prehistoric times and are natural constituents of the fish that possess them. Probably the best-known example is the Japanese fugu, a variety of puffer, which is considered a delicacy among its aficionados. Though licensed handlers are required to have a knowledge of the

Common Fishes Responsible for Marine Food Poisoning

Poison	Common name of fish responsible	Habitat
ciguatoxin	grouper	Caribbean, Indo-Pacific
	jack	Caribbean
	pompano	Caribbean
	red snapper	Tropical Pacific
clupleotoxin*	anchovy	Peru and Chile
	herring	Caribbean to Cape Cod
	sardine	Indo-Pacific and Malaya
tetradotoxin	puffer	Tropical seas, China, Japan, Pacific and Atlantic coasts of U.S.

*similar to cigua

Source: Graham: *The Safety of Foods.*[48]

toxic species, several hundred poisoning cases are recorded in Japan each year, and about half of them are fatal.

Although the fugu enthusiast knows the risk involved and pursues his passion despite (or because of) its danger, the unsuspecting consumer may be liable to poisoning by toxic varieties of a number of fairly common types of fish. Though these need not be a deterrent to the use of other good-quality seafood, it behooves the fish-eater to inform himself about the varieties that are likely to be toxic so he can avoid them. Illness can result from eating the flesh or certain organs or eggs of approximately 500 saltwater species. Fortunately, only a small percentage of these types of fish are commonly consumed by humans. (See table on p. 164.) But in these cases, catching or buying the wrong variety can lead to serious consequences.

Though a number of these fish toxins are known, the major public health hazard is ciguatera poisoning. The cigua toxin produces a tingling and numbness about the lips, followed by

Guidelines for Fish Consumption

1. Buy fish from reputable, large supermarkets that are likely to require their suppliers to be certified, or from fish markets where you can establish some rapport and learn about their sources. Watch for evidence that fish is allowed to thaw and be refrozen.

2. Stick with deep-water seafish when possible. Be wary of odd varieties from small suppliers that could carry natural fish toxins.

3. Be sure shellfish are well cooked and, if possible, that they come from approved waters.

4. Use the same precautions in handling raw seafoods, especially shellfish, as you would in handling raw poultry or meat (see previous two chapters of this book).

5. If fish or shellfish don't look and smell fresh and appealing, don't buy them. (Have tofu instead for dinner that night!)

6. If you live in an area with waters that are known to be polluted, keep abreast of local conditions and current reports on the levels of contaminants in fish caught nearby.

nausea, abdominal cramps, and pain. Although there is a usually progressive weakness that can go as far as paralysis, convulsions, and even death, less than 1 case in 10 is in fact fatal. No effective treatment is available. It has been estimated that about 2,000 outbreaks of ciguatera poisoning occur in and around the Pacific each year. Certain species of red snapper, pompano, jackfish, groupers, and eels carry the toxin.[48]

Serious poisoning can also result from eating shellfish that have fed on certain plankton containing a toxic substance. Paralytic shellfish poisoning, as it is called, is similar to cigua toxicity in symptoms and mortality rate and has been acquired by eating clams, mussels, scallops, and crabs.

If, on the basis of all the evidence presented, one decides to omit fish from the diet, he must be sure that he does not, by removing all animal foods from the diet, fail to provide the one essential nutrient that is not present in plant foods: vitamin B_{12}.

VITAMIN B_{12} AND PERNICIOUS ANEMIA

Probably no nutrient is so indelibly stamped on the mind of the vegetarian as B_{12}. It is often said that a vegetarian diet can supply everything but this vitamin. Physicians and nutritionists are trained to caution those who are eliminating all animal foods about the grave consequences of B_{12} deficiency and to advise them that, at the very least, B_{12} supplements should be taken. This concern is understandable. Pernicious anemia, the dread disease connected with insufficient body stores of vitamin B_{12}, is enough to give anyone pause.

The pernicious anemia patient was first described in the medical literature in 1849 as one who appeared pale and sallow with a shiny tongue and complained of weakness and fatigue that progressed gradually to the point of paralysis. Blood tests done on such patients today would reveal low hemoglobin levels and large, pale, red blood cells. In the early stages of the illness there are numbness and tingling in the hands and feet with a loss of sensation. Gradually a lack of motor coordination develops. These symptoms are now known to be due to an inability to synthesize myelin, the fatty sheath that insulates nerve fibers. As a result, the nerves to the limbs degenerate. If allowed to proceed unchecked, the deterioration progresses into the spinal cord and ultimately to the brain. Moodiness, poor memory, and confusion give way gradually to delusions, hallucinations, and overt psychosis.

A genetic predisposition has been observed, the typical patient being described as tall and blue-eyed, with large ears and premature greying of the hair. The incidence of the disease in Caucasians of northern European stock is thought to be a little over 1 per 1,000, and approaches 1 in 100 in the over-60 age group.[49] Recently, such patients have been shown to produce antibodies against their own gastric lining cells, so it is thought that the disease may have an auto-immune basis.

For B_{12} to be absorbed, the stomach wall must secrete a substance called intrinsic factor, which combines with the B_{12}, forming a complex that can then be taken up by the lower end of the small intestine. Patients with pernicious anemia were found to lack intrinsic factor because of the destruction of stomach wall cells. Thus B_{12}, even when present in the diet in ample quantities, cannot be absorbed.

When originally described, the disease was observed to occur sporadically in most populations without regard to dietary practices. It was not considered to result from inadequate dietary intake of B_{12}. Indeed there was no reason to assume that the disease had anything to do with the amount of vitamin B_{12} consumed, since amounts many times that ordinarily needed are of no use without intrinsic factor.

Nevertheless, because it has long been known that vitamin B_{12} is absent from foods that are strictly of plant origin, when nutritionists and dieticians began to encounter growing numbers of strict vegetarians, they were alarmed. While vegetarians who used dairy products were generally thought to be on safe ground,[50-52] vegans, who take no foods of animal origin, were a different matter. A diet with no B_{12}, it was felt, was sure to produce B_{12} deficiency and, ultimately, pernicious anemia.

Dietary Deficiency of B_{12}: Myth or Reality?

In the 1960s and 1970s a large number of case reports in medical journals seemed to fulfill this dire prophecy: "Subacute combined degeneration of the spinal cord in a vegan,"[53] "Megaloblastic anemia in an adult vegan,"[54] and so on. Nutrition manuals warned of the danger of developing pernicious anemia from an inadequate intake of vitamin B_{12}.[55] But despite the ominous tone of such case reports, surveys of groups of vegans reported with some surprise that most of the subjects they studied seemed quite well, with no signs of anemia or neurological degeneration. The occurrence of symptoms was, at most, rare.[52,56] One might expect, after all, to find some cases of the disease in any population.

Were the cases of pernicious anemia that were reported merely persons with the disease who happened to be vegans, or were these cases caused by the all-plant diet? Of course, vegans argued the former in their magazines and newsletters, while nutritionists argued the latter in their books and scientific journals. As is usual with such debates, the ardor of the controversy yielded little in the way of illumination.

Nevertheless, by the beginning of the 1980s there was enough published literature to make evident some of the oversights that had led to premature conclusions: many of the diagnoses of inadequate B_{12} in the diet had been hastily made. For example, problems that can interfere with absorption, such as a lack of intrinsic factor, had not been ruled out as causes of the low body levels of B_{12}. To establish firmly that a person is suffering from a *dietary* deficiency of vitamin B_{12}, certain criteria must be met.[nt.7]

A critical review of reports published up to 1980 on vegans showed that none of them met all these criteria.[52] In each case, other explanations were possible, including deficiency of intrinsic factor, iron deficiency anemia, and neurological problems from other causes. In fact, in many of the published case reports, the authors noted that these alternative explanations seemed the most likely. Yet the cumulative weight of the first impressions created by numbers of such scientific papers is persuasive in itself and has tended to support the view not only that dietary deficiency of B_{12} is an actuality, but that it is common among vegetarians who use no animal foods. Despite this prevailing impression, in point of fact there is little incontrovertible evidence that a diet low in B_{12} can, in and of itself, cause problems.[nt.8]

B_{12} *Vegan Sources*

If it's true that a purely dietary deficiency of B_{12} occurs rarely, if at all, the question is, Why? How could it be that vegans, who consistently consume no B_{12}-containing foods at all, might be perfectly healthy, with adequate tissue levels of the vitamin?

At least part of the answer to this question becomes apparent when we look at the origin of vitamin B_{12}. Though it is found in animal foods, it is not manufactured by animal cells. It must be absorbed from their food by most animals, as it must be by humans. All B_{12} is made by bacteria. Ruminants, such as cows, do quite well, because bacteria in an accessory stomach, or rumen, produce B_{12} as they break down the fiber of the animal's food. But bacteria aren't just in cows' stomachs; they're practically everywhere. Researchers studying B_{12} have complained that it's necessary to carefully clean all instruments to get meaningful measurements of B_{12}, since even tap water can contain substantial amounts. (At least these amounts are substantial in the sense that they can approach the range of what is needed in the human diet.)

It is for this reason that some batches of beans, bean sprouts, comfrey leaves, turnip greens, peanuts, lettuce, fermented soybeans, and whole wheat have been reported to contain significant levels of B_{12}—while other batches of the same foods have been found to have none at all. The presence of bacteria on such foods is incidental; that is, the presence or absence of the vitamin will depend on whether the plants were fertilized with manure or not, how well they were washed and with what, and so forth. So as sources of B_{12} any one of such foods must be considered unreliable, though on any average day several of them might happen to bring along some small but significant amounts of B_{12}.

What's more, bacteria also grow on and in the body. In fact, it has been estimated that the microorganisms between the teeth and gums, around and in the crevices of the tonsils, in the folds at the base of the tongue, and in the upper respiratory passages will make up to half a microgram of B_{12} a day.[59] This is at least half of the minimum requirement, though some nutritionists think this quantity may be all that is needed for most people. Official recommended intakes by the World Health Organization and the Food and Nutrition Board provide for generous margins of safety, and up the level to as high as 3 or 4 micrograms for adults, but it is unlikely that it is necessary or even useful to consume such large amounts. An egg or a cup of milk will contain 1 microgram of B_{12} (see table below).

Microecology of the Gut

There are countless bacteria in the human intestinal tract, too. Whether or not they make a contribution to the B_{12} needs of their

B_{12} Content of Common Foods

Food	Amount	B_{12} (mcg)
Organ meats (e.g., liver)	3 oz	>10
Bivalves (clams, oysters)	3 oz	>10
Milk	1 cup	1
Fish	3 oz	1-3
Beef	3 oz	1-3
Chicken	3 oz	1-3
Cheese, hard	1 oz	0.3
Egg yolk	1	1
Fermented soy products: Miso Tempeh	 1 T 3 oz	 c. 0.03 (variable) c. 3 (variable)
Seaweed	—	variable
Spirulina*	—	variable
Yogurt	1 c	0.3

*See p. 174.

Sources: Goodman & Gillman: *Pharmacological Basis of Therapeutics.*[60] U.S. Dept. of Agriculture: *Vitamin B$_{12}$ in Foods.*[61] Shurtleff: *Sources of B$_{12}$.*[62]

human host is a subject of another long-standing controversy. Early studies on the bacterial flora of the gut focused on the colon, where the bulk of the intestinal microorganisms are found. The discovery that many of these bacteria were producers of B_{12} led to the rather hasty conclusion that this B_{12} would pass through the wall of the large intestine and serve as a major source of the vitamin. One researcher, while pessimistic about the vegan's chances of avoiding serious neurological disease, allowed that "a water extract of one's own feces contains enough B_{12} to treat a deficiency," but noted that studies show it's not absorbed from the colon,[63] implying perhaps that using it in any fashion at all would present hygienic and aesthetic problems of major proportions.

A new light was thrown on the question, however, when more refined research techniques revealed that a smaller but still substantial community of bacteria inhabits the small intestine. Recent studies have demonstrated that these organisms do produce B_{12} and that they do so high enough in the intestinal tract to allow it to combine with intrinsic factor before it reaches the lower end of the small intestine, where the vitamin is absorbed.[64]

It had been observed that South Indian vegans migrating to England not infrequently developed symptoms of B_{12} deficiency. In India the problem had been practically nonexistent among these same people, although they had followed an all-plant diet there too. Why this should be so was not clear. But when the bacterial population of the small intestines of healthy South Indians was studied, it was found to be more extensive than that of Britishers. On the basis of such evidence researchers hypothesized that the number and types of bacteria colonizing the intestines of those living in India may have been able to manufacture sufficient B_{12} to prevent deficiency, but that the shift in intestinal ecology occurring with immigration had resulted in a scantier and less productive bacterial population and insufficient B_{12} to meet the vegans' needs. Losing their own internal B_{12} factory, they had developed B_{12} deficiency symptoms.[nt.9]

Another complication is that some bacteria will compete with their host for dietary B_{12} without contributing significant quantities in return. They can even deplete body stores, since B_{12} is constantly being secreted with the bile. Though ordinarily much of this is reabsorbed as the bile passes through the intestinal tract, bacteria with an inclination for robbing their host of vitamins have a clear shot at this B_{12}. But in one who has a well-balanced, "friendly" population of microbes in the intestinal tract, the B_{12} that is excreted in the bile can be reabsorbed almost entirely, so that little is lost from the body in the feces, and dietary needs for B_{12} are reduced.

It's also known that B_{12} absorption is more thorough when intake is lower. In other words, the meat-eater who consumes 10 micrograms of B_{12} in a day will absorb only 16% of it, while the vegan, who takes in a mere fraction of that (perhaps one half a microgram), will absorb 70% of it.[65]

Probably it is for all these reasons that a healthy vegan can remain healthy without fish, milk, or any other animal foods. With his intake of traces of bacteria in his food, with his oral, pharyngeal, and intestinal production of B_{12}, with his thorough recycling of B_{12} from the bile, and with a high rate of absorption of the multiple small quantities of B_{12} that reach his lower small intestine, he manages quite well. He has a smoothly working system that is efficient and effective. Everything will be fine as long as nothing happens to disrupt the balance of his B_{12} production and utilization.

Although it is now clear why vegans are generally able to do quite well as far as B_{12} goes, the next question is, Why are there some who don't? Published reports show that there are a few, though apparently not many, who do run into some sort of trouble. Why would these vegans, taking the same all-plant diet as their healthy counterparts, become B_{12} deficient? There are two basic answers: either their absorption of the relatively small amounts of B_{12} they have available is compromised, or their needs are increased. A disturbance in the microecology of the intestine due to some major disruption such as migration or the use of antibiotic medications[66] is one of the events that can tip this delicate balance. Others that are important:

1. Excess fat or protein. Too much of either in the diet can increase B_{12} needs.

2. Highly processed foods. Whereas boiling milk for two to five minutes only decreased its B_{12} content by 30%, sterilization in sealed containers for 13 minutes caused a loss of 77%.[63] Canned milk, for example, might be inadequate as a source of B_{12}.

3. Drugs. Tobacco, alcohol, coffee, and birth control pills have all been implicated in increasing one's needs for B_{12}.[59]

4. Pregnancy and nursing. Both pregnancy and nursing increase B_{12} needs. Low intake during nursing, for example, has resulted in breastmilk that is deficient even when the mother's levels remain normal,[67,68] and has also resulted in symptoms such as apathy and retardation in the infant.[69]

5. Chronic disease. Intestinal parasites, malaria, liver disease, chronic infections, and cancer will all disrupt normal mechanisms of B_{12} absorption and use, and increase needs.

6. Intestinal surgery. Removal of part of the stomach, where intrinsic factor is made and secreted, or removal of part of the lower small intestine, where it is absorbed, can drastically reduce uptake and may necessitate the use of injectable B_{12}.

7. Use of megadoses of vitamin C, multiple vitamin/mineral preparations containing copper, and perhaps other food supplements such as spirulina (see below).

B_{12}, Mega C, and Other Supplements

Another ongoing controversy is that surrounding the effects of large doses of vitamin C on B_{12} availability. In 1974, one of the most respected authorities on vitamin B_{12} reported that mixing vitamin C with vitamin B_{12} and incubating the combination in a way that would mimic digestion destroyed B_{12}.[70] Both the popular news media and the medical literature were quickly filled with warnings about the danger of vitamin C. Two years later, however, a different author observed that the original study had been done using methods of B_{12} measurement that were designed to test blood, not food. Since the B_{12} in food is more tightly bound to proteins, he concluded that the tests used had failed to pick it up. Using more appropriate techniques, no destruction of B_{12} was found.[71] The researcher who had done the first study retaliated in 1978, demonstrating low blood levels of B_{12} in patients who took 2 grams of vitamin C a day and noting that another study had reported similar results.[72]

Although the issue is still not completely resolved, it would appear that anyone taking more than 500 milligrams of vitamin C daily for a long period of time should have his or her vitamin B_{12} status monitored. An alternative that might provide some protection is to take vitamin C in high doses only for short periods of time, allowing intervals when it is stopped so that B_{12} stores can be replenished. A convenient regimen is one week on and one week off.

But other nutritional supplements can cause trouble, too. It is well established that B_{12} is destroyed by oxygen in the presence of vitamin C, vitamin B_1(thiamine), and copper ions. This may affect the B_{12} present in multivitamin preparations. It has been reported that 20% to 90% of the vitamin present in such supplements can be degraded to B_{12} analogues.[73] These are B_{12}-like molecules that are similar enough to the real thing to replace it in metabolic reactions, but different enough to lack the effectiveness of the vitamin.[74] Some of them can thus block the activity of the B_{12} that is present, preventing it from being used normally.[73]

Spirulina, a dietary supplement widely acclaimed as an extraordinary source of B_{12}, has also been found to contain much more B_{12} analogues than genuine B_{12}—five to eight times as much.[75] Whether or not these analogues are B_{12} antagonists and cause harm awaits investigation.

B_{12} as an oral supplement, when taken separately from other nutrients that can degrade it, such as vitamin C, copper, and thiamine, can be of help, however. It can be used by those with inadequate dietary B_{12} or when illness may increase one's needs beyond what is a normally adequate dietary intake. It can even be effective in those cases where absorption is impaired by a lack of intrinsic factor, since somewhere between 1% and 3% of vitamin B_{12} passes across the intestinal wall by simple diffusion.[65] But much higher doses must be used when the normal mechanisms of active uptake are missing. Under these circumstances 75 to 100 micrograms must be taken to ensure a significant intake. In severe cases of B_{12} depletion, it is usually considered safer to use an injectable form of the vitamin.

Nutritional yeast is sometimes used as a dietary supplement to supply vitamin B_{12} by those who are consuming only vegetable foods. Not all nutritional or brewer's yeast, however, will furnish the vitamin. In order to contain B_{12} the medium on which such yeast is grown must contain it or it must be added during the final processing. If one wishes to use yeast as a source, one must read labels carefully to be sure that the yeast in question does indeed contain the vitamin, and in adequate amounts (at least 1 microgram in 1 tablespoon, since a tablespoonful is a maximal appropriate regular daily dose of yeast[nt.10]).

MEAL PLANNING: ESCAPING THE ENTREE MENTALITY

The elimination of fish from the diet will bring one to a new stage in one's perspectives on eating patterns. As long as fish remained, it was logical and comfortable to organize the meals around an entree. In nonvegetarian diets it is the steak, the ham, the chicken dish, or the fish that serves as the focus of the meal. The other components of the menu, such as vegetables, grains,

---

What to Do About B_{12}

1. If you use substantial amounts of fish, milk, or eggs, you have an extra margin of safety. If not:

2. Don't smoke, drink coffee, use alcohol regularly, or take birth control pills.

3. Beware of the use of antibiotics or contaminated meat, poultry, or fish that can create havoc in the microbial population of the intestinal tract.

4. If you develop an illness, especially a chronic one, pay particular attention to your B_{12} intake, or better yet, find a physician knowledgeable about nutrition to help.

potatoes, or salad, are organized around this central feature that is thought of as the main dish. Budding vegetarians often try to hang on to what's familiar by substituting "vegetarian entrees" such as eggplant parmigiana, spinach quiche, or cheese soufflé. These are not true vegetarian meals, but really cheese or eggs substituted for meat.

But of course the vegetarians of the world have not resigned themselves wistfully to a lifetime of meals that are missing their main dish. The best of vegetarian meals are organized in a completely different fashion. In order to understand this, we must examine the reasons for having an entree.

In meat meals, the meat brings several important features nutritionally. It supplies protein, minerals, and taste appeal. It is usually the most concentrated and substantial part of the meal. In fact, it is so concentrated and so substantial that it relies on other components of the meal to balance it by being milder, fresher, lighter, and of a totally different nature. Eliminating the meat, fowl, or fish entree then leaves the meal "empty," and one feels the necessity of filling this emptiness with some substitute, such as an omelette, a dish rich in cheese, or perhaps a meat analogue, one of the vegetable protein products designed to fill the spot usually occupied by an animal food entree.

In the vegetarian menu, the features present in the animal food entree may be scattered through several dishes or contained in any one of a number of them. For example, the bean dish in a vegetarian meal, such as baked beans, may be very meaty and substitute for the usual entree. Even so, however, it is not as concentrated or as substantial as meat, and one finds it quite pleasing to have along with this bean dish a rather substantial, heavy, whole-grain bread. Thus, the Boston tradition of baked beans and brown bread.

For the sake of comparison, a meal that combines both meat and whole-grain bread is rather too much, and meat-lovers are usually those who favor lighter and whiter bread. On the other hand, bean dishes can be made rather light, and the substance of the meal can be concentrated more in the vegetable dish. A preparation containing fried onions, mushrooms, and cooked-

down string beans, for example, can be quite meaty and substantial. In this case a light dish made of white rice and split,
hulled, mung beans can provide a pleasing contrast.

Many variations are possible. Though the ethnic cuisines of
people around the world who follow low-meat diets provide many
inspiring examples, we would do well to remember that most of
them are neither purely vegetarian nor intentionally so. Their
meatless meals are used to tide the family over during seasons of
meat shortage, or are modifications of meat meals that seize on
available ingredients in order to increase the palatability of what is
regarded as second-rate food. Such dietary practices, evolved out
of economic necessity, may often be ingenious in their ability to
make the best nutritional use of what's at hand, but they are
unlikely to be optimal.

Although as a new vegetarianism takes shape it will draw on
traditions from all over the world, it is those that have most
thoroughly integrated the principles of good nutrition that will
prove to be most valuable. Ethnic diets that are based partly on
meat, and use meatless meals only occasionally, when economic
considerations dictate, are unlikely to offer as useful a model as
those that have been consistently vegetarian.

From this perspective the classical vegetarian cuisine of India
is of unique interest. It evolved among a group of people that
was educated, relatively affluent, and intent on devising a meatless diet that would be both healthful and conducive to alertness
and clarity of consciousness. Indian vegetarian cuisine also had
a vast store of traditional knowledge about the properties of
herbs and spices from which to draw. The result is a cuisine
whose subtlety, elegance, and sophistication are only now beginning to be appreciated in the West.[nt.11]

One indication that a diet is oriented toward good vegetarian
nutrition is a thorough and skillful integration of legumes into the
overall fabric of the diet. Classical Indian vegetarian dishes include
legumes in a wide variety of forms, such as breads, crisp papad,
soups, sauces, dahls, and even desserts. Distributing the protein
and the flavor appeal through a number of dishes in the meal
means that each of them is satisfying in and of itself. The Indian

vegetarian *thali* or platter with its assortment of little bowls, each containing an individual serving of some dish based on vegetables, beans, or grains (or a combination thereof), probably represents the most thorough possible escape from the entree mentality.

Other indications of an evolved approach to vegetarian eating crop up in this tradition, too. For example, the chewy, satisfying texture that meats usually furnish is provided for here by flat breads that are unique in their substance and texture. There is an incredible variety of them, chapatis and paranthas being the best known to Westerners. Part of their appeal may also come from the fact that they expose the wheat to an intensity of heat that is thought to increase its digestibility and eliminate some of its disadvantages. Although this is another area that has not been studied, it is the present author's clinical observation that most people experience less heaviness and more alertness after a meal of whole-wheat chapati than of whole-wheat yeasted bread.

Classical Indian cuisine might justifiably be expected to provide the more adventurous and imaginative of modern nutritionists with a wealth of hypotheses as research on vegetarianism becomes more sophisticated and more oriented toward the study of the details of the practical application of the principles that are now emerging. The best of Indian meatless cooking should also serve as a major inspiration for a new generation of vegetarians.

But not all Indian ethnic cuisine is worthy of emulation. Economic necessity, changes in the availability of basic foodstuffs, and the invasion of foreign influences have all taken their toll and contributed to the corruption of the ideal. A diet of potatoes, cauliflower, and eggplant, drenched in oil and ablaze with chili peppers, is nearly the antithesis of the sattvic diet advocated by the classical writers on yoga and Ayurveda. North Indian cuisine, at least that of certain Himalayan areas, has perhaps remained the purest example of an intentionally optimal vegetarian diet.

The recipe on the following page is adapted from a style of cooking followed by Himalayan monks who are exposed to a climate similar to that of temperate North America, and who thus need food of some substance, but who are also attuned to the effects of food on health and consciousness, and thus especially

Himalayan Mountain Bread

1-1/2 cup whole-wheat flour

1 package yeast

4 oz water or whey

1/2 tsp. sugar

1-1/2 cup leftover mashed beans

2/3 cup pureed peeled tomato (optional)

3 T flaked blanched almonds

3 T broken cashews

3 T white raisins

8 oz shredded mozarella

salt

butter for oiling skillet

    Mix 2 oz hot water in a cup with the sugar. Add yeast. Allow yeast to froth, then add with rest of liquid to flour. Knead briefly, then pat or roll out. Lay in a greased 12″ heavy cast-iron skillet, and set over low flame (for 5 minutes while rest of ingredients are added). Press dough until it fills bottom of pan evenly and has a 1/2″ raised edge. Sprinkle with salt, nuts, and raisins. Spoon beans over this and spread evenly with a rubber spatula. If tomato is used, pour it on and then cover thinly with cheese. Bake at 350° for about 20 minutes (until cheese is golden brown and bread pulls away from edges of pan). Slice, pizza-style, and serve with beans and rice, a cooked green vegetable, and a green salad.

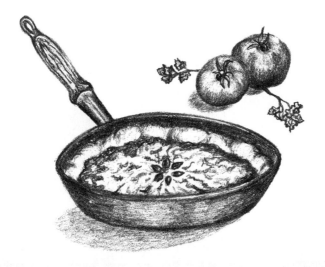

attentive to traditional dietary guidelines. A wide variety of authentic recipes in this tradition have been detailed elsewhere.[81]

By the end of Phase 3 one should have established what is a basically sound vegetarian diet. In the next chapter we will discuss the final refinements of this diet that can further its ability to provide good health, and that may even extend life and ensure alertness into old age.

Goals for Phase 3

1. To have eliminated:

- red meat
- refined sugars
- fowl
- refined flour
- **unreliable, unsafe sources of fish**
- **raw or undercooked shellfish. Use knowledgeably selected fish three to five times a week, or eliminate all fish and use milk products and eggs instead.**

2. To have added:

- a grain/legume combination **three to four times a week**
- a fresh, cooked, leafy green vegetable at least **three to four times a week**

3. To take regularly:

- two pieces of fresh fruit each day
- a green salad once a day
- a fresh, cooked, green or yellow vegetable each day
- **two** servings of whole grains **each day**

NOW THAT YOU'RE A VEGETARIAN

MILK AND EGGS

It could be argued that, in the strictest sense, one is not vegetarian until he or she has eliminated all animal foods of all sorts. In the West, however, vegetarianism is most often understood to include the consumption of milk and eggs. But the use of the term varies and there are those who refer to themselves as vegetarian even though they eat some fish. This need not be as much of a contradiction as it seems. Consistent with what we have learned so far in this book about a healthful vegetarian diet, it may make sense to consider one who takes fish a vegetarian if such a person follows a diet of primarily fresh, cooked green vegetables, fresh fruits, and grain/legume combinations, supplemented with small amounts of fish. But if one follows a conventional diet of the sort that is ordinarily organized around meat and poultry, and merely substitutes fish and other seafoods for the meat entrees, then that person is not a vegetarian in any sense of the word. Instead, he or she is a meat-eater who only happens to eat the meat of marine animals rather than that of land animals.

This is more than a semantic distinction. If the diet is sound, relying for its basic constituents on good-quality plant foods, in the combinations and proportions that typify the diets of peoples who eat little or no meat and maintain good health, then it might properly be considered a vegetarian diet. In fact, there is no compelling reason why it should not.

The origin of the term "vegetarian" can be traced to the Latin *vegetare,* which means "to enliven." This is related to *vegere* and *vigere,* which mean "to arouse" and "to flourish." From the latter also come "vigorous" and "vigil," which connotes wakeful or alert. The most ancient root word is *wag,* to be lively or strong. The basis of the term "vegetarian," then, is a sense of liveliness, vigor, and alertness, rather than merely an indication of a diet of vegetables. The issue is not whether the diet is or isn't made up exclusively of foods of plant origins (vegetable foods) but whether it is enlivening and health-giving. What is used as a supplemental source of protein and other nutrients, be it milk, eggs, fish, or even fowl or meat, is a less important consideration.

But if these supplemental protein foods become major constituents of the diet, then they begin to affect the health and consciousness of those who consume them, both by virtue of their own properties as well as through the effects they have on the sort of foods that tend to be selected to accompany them. Hence as we have observed, heavy meat-eaters tend to prefer white bread, lightly cooked vegetables, and sweets as complements and counterbalances to their meat.

Supplemental protein foods, even when taken in small amounts, can also come to play a dominant role in the diet if their quality is so poor that they carry a substantial risk for serious disease. Thus, even small amounts of beef or poultry, if contaminated with antibiotic-resistant microbes, have no place in a diet or a kitchen that is *vegetare,* life-giving.

It might also be maintained that supplemental foods come to dominate and transform a diet if they have negative effects on consciousness. If the physiological effects of a relatively small amount of meat are such that they stimulate a pointless hostile aggressiveness or a chronic low level of fear and anxiety, one might feel justified in concluding that the diet has lost its vegetarian essence and that it is no longer appropriate to apply that term to it.

Of course, as noted earlier, insofar as modern scientific investigations are concerned, such effects of diet have not been studied. Nevertheless, since the possibility of important mental and emotional repercussions from diet should not be overlooked, it may seem appropriate to have recourse to traditional teachings and the principles set forth by those who based their conclusions on introspective observation.

From these traditions come concepts such as that of *ahimsa,* or nonviolence. In the East the cultivation of this quality is considered not so much a moral imperative as it is a device designed to unburden or enliven one's consciousness.

Though the modern shopper picking up a neatly wrapped package of meat from a supermarket display case might feel quite remote from feedlots and slaughterhouses, the origin of his food is not unknown to him, and Eastern concepts of psychological functioning which see each action as bringing into the unconscious mind a whole set of consequent associations and images are not out of keeping with more modern ideas of how the mind works. From this perspective the mental field would become progressively cluttered with the reverberations of eating habits that require the abuse and slaughter of animals. Such psychological and emotional effects would, on some level, and to some extent, dissipate mental energy and distract attention, and would as a result be considered a handicap and a hindrance to full alertness and clarity of consciousness. One aspect of the philosophies on which such psychological insights are based is the priority given to clarity of consciousness. It is seen not only as a prerequisite to the discovery of the aim of one's life, but also as critical for the attainment of such an aim.

Through painstaking and persistent self-scrutiny the sages of ancient times catalogued those influences that could distract and disrupt consciousness. Flesh foods aroused the animal instincts of aggression and fear, they concluded. On the other hand, milk and eggs (at least those not fertilized) created different effects. They are nourishment given to the young. They do not require the taking of life; their essence is, on the contrary, the giving of life. They could easily be accepted in that spirit—as a gift, given by nature to nourish and to nurture.

Whether or not one feels sympathy with such a perspective,

according to time-honored usage vegetarians do not consume meat, fowl, or fish, though they may well consume milk and perhaps eggs. (Technically speaking, and in order to avoid ambiguity, one who takes vegetable foods, dairy products, and eggs is an ovolactovegetarian.) Probably the largest concentration of long-term vegetarians in the world is found on the Indian subcontinent, where the precepts of psychological and spiritual development just described had a major impact on the evolution of cultural patterns among the masses. There, the term vegetarian is generally assumed to mean one who uses milk products, though most often this does not include the use of eggs. Such people of course are correctly labeled lactovegetarians.

The percentage of vegetarians in the world who are vegans is quite small. They not only avoid both milk and eggs, many of them strictly avoid all foods that are in any sense animal products, such as honey. As we have seen, it is among these people that deficiency states are most likely to occur and that the diet must be most closely regulated. Without the supplemental protein that could come from fish or milk and eggs, one must keep a watchful eye on protein quality and quantity. This is especialy true with growing children and adolescents. Vitamin B_{12} is, as mentioned in the previous chapter, another matter to be watched carefully. Riboflavin, vitamin B_2, is also more of a problem for the vegan than for the lactovegetarian, since milk is a good source of it.

Milk is not particularly rich in zinc and is actually a rather poor source of iron, but the vegan may have more trouble with these nutrients than the lactovegetarian does, simply because his fiber intake is likely to be twice as high. Because of this, he runs the risk of pushing his intake of phytates and other mineral-binding substances beyond what can be adapted to, and as a result may absorb inadequate amounts of these minerals. Calcium is also of concern to the vegan because, though it is plentiful in milk and milk products, it is not so plentiful in many vegetable foods. Green leafy vegetables can help the vegan supply his calcium needs, but without milk products vegetarians who get little sunshine for long periods may also have problems with vitamin D, as we have seen, and have difficulty absorbing the calcium they eat.

In view of all the problems they can help one avoid, why would one wish to eliminate milk products and eggs? One consideration is hygienic. Many of the complications arising from modern live-stock management that have undermined the quality of meat and poultry are also having adverse effects on milk and eggs. The quality of both products has declined in recent decades, as can be seen quite graphically in the case of eggs.

Most eggs today are mass-produced. Laying hens are generally housed four or five to a 12" x 18" cage. Food and water are brought in mechanically and eggs are removed the same way. Through selective breeding and careful formulation of feeds, productivity has been pushed to the point that each hen lays an egg two out of every three days. Conditions are so unnatural that the birds' behavior is disturbed and they must be debeaked to prevent them from pecking each other to death. In addition, their bones grad-ually decalcify as a result of inactivity. The hens suffer not only from overcrowding but also from other stresses. The wire floor of the cage, for example, designed to let droppings fall through, is made of wire that is spaced so far apart as to provide little support. As a result, the birds' feet, suited to perching on limbs or scratching in the earth, must cause them constant distress. Un-der these conditions, the hens generally last only a couple of years before their productivity falls off. Eggs produced under such circumstances are unlikely to provide a very healthful source of food.

One solution to the problem of egg quality is to simply eliminate eggs from the diet. Another is to seek out eggs that have been produced under better conditions. Marketed under a special label ("Nest Eggs" is an example), these eggs come from hens that are allowed to run free and that are fed a diet that has no chemical additives or pesticides. Such eggs, though usually more expensive, are, according to the growers, more wholesome—higher in B_{12}, for example—and noticeably tastier. However, even with the best of eggs, there remains the matter of cholesterol.

Eggs and Cholesterol

Technically, cholesterol is not a fat. It is a waxy sort of substance with a complex and unusual molecular structure that most closely resembles certain hormones that are often manufactured from it. (See figure below.) Though necessary as a raw material for the manufacture of such hormones, as well as of vitamin D and bile acids, and though present in the body in relatively small amounts, cholesterol nonetheless gained notoriety because of its presence in atherosclerotic plaques. When it was first noticed that deposits were largely cholesterol, it was understandably assumed that reducing cholesterol in the diet might prevent the deposit of cholesterol in the arteries, thereby reducing the frequency of heart attacks and strokes. High-cholesterol foods such as meats, eggs, and dairy products, previously coveted as dietary mainstays, were suddenly seen in a negative light, and a campaign to reduce their use ensued.

Of course, the finding of cholesterol in the arteries doesn't

Important Derivatives of Cholesterol

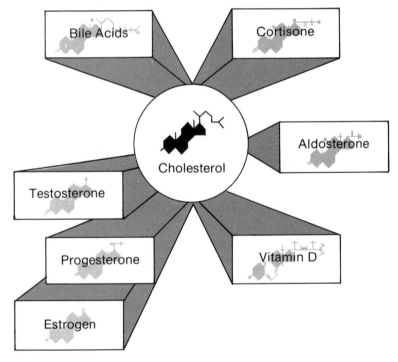

Source: Brisson: *Lipids in Human Nutrition.*[1]

necessarily mean it came from the diet. Indeed, research showed that the body manufactures its own cholesterol and if dietary intake is low enough, it makes more. This was good news for the egg industry, and scrambled eggs were back on the breakfast table. But further research suggested that the physiological mechanisms for the adjustment of cholesterol levels might have their limitations. If dietary cholesterol were quite high, perhaps the body wouldn't be able to cut back production enough to keep levels of cholesterol from rising. So, exit eggs, once again.

Next came the revelation that eggs contain a substance that helps keep cholesterol in solution. This substance, lecithin, it was suggested, decreases cholesterol's tendency to settle out and form solid masses such as the deposits in the arteries or gallstones (which are, as it turns out, largely crystallized cholesterol). Now not only were eggs back on the breakfast table again, the whole meal was likely to be sprinkled with granular lecithin!

And so it has gone. From revelation to counterrevelation, the controversy has raged on, fueled by political and economic interests and illuminated by the uncertain light of half-truths. Research studies have been quoted (and misquoted) to prove that eggs raise blood cholesterol[2] or that they don't.[3-6] And called into question in the process is the actual significance of blood cholesterol levels. Do they really matter anyhow? Are they in fact related to heart disease?

Dietary Cholesterol and Heart Disease

Even when research shows a statistical correlation between two events, that doesn't mean one causes the other. For example, studies done on cholesterol in the diet and heart disease in many countries can be summarized graphically (see figure on p. 190). There is a strong general tendency for heart disease rates to be higher in countries where cholesterol consumption is quite high, like the U.S.A. and New Zealand, when compared with countries that have diets very low in cholesterol, like Japan and Italy, though in the middle range, where intake is moderate, that is not true.[nt.1]

But this doesn't mean that cholesterol consumption is the

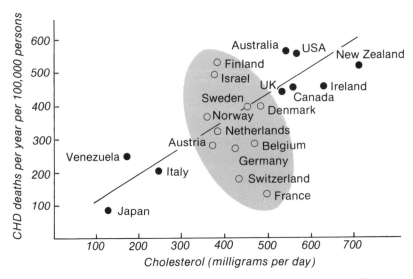

Relationships Between Dietary Cholesterol and Mortality from Coronary Heart Disease (CHD)

Source: Brisson: *Lipids in Human Nutrition.*[7]

cause of the heart disease. In fact, some maintain that dietary cholesterol has nothing to do with heart disease at all. Though the correlation seems too dramatic to be dismissed entirely, there is the strong possibility that a high cholesterol level in the diet functions primarily as a marker, indicating the presence of other causative factors in diet or lifestyle.

As it turns out, this probably is the principal significance of high levels of cholesterol in the diet. Those countries with higher cholesterol intake also eat more meat, which as we saw in Phase 1 has been found to be associated with an increased rate of death from heart disease. They eat more total fat and oil, too, another good candidate for a major causative role in heart disease. And they smoke more.[7] So cholesterol-rich diets may simply flag populations that are at high risk for heart disease because of other things they do.

The whole issue has remained unnecessarily complex and confusing. This is most likely due to the difficulty of studying a disease like atherosclerosis, which is so universal in our population and provoked by so many factors, such as high dietary meat and fat, smoking, lack of exercise, and trace mineral deficiencies, all of which are also common. When many of these causes are acting in concert to produce a disease that affects practically everybody, altering only one of them is unlikely to produce a very dramatic effect. So even if cholesterol intake were playing some role in the development of the disease, research studies involving changes in cholesterol consumption in this context probably wouldn't show it.

In any case, a careful review of literature in the field[8,9] yields a few fairly safe conclusions. First, people respond differently: when 21 healthy middle-aged men were given an extra three eggs a day for a month, 8 of them showed increases in blood cholesterol that were quite significant. The other 13 experienced no increase in blood cholesterol levels on the extra eggs, and this held true for half of them even when their egg intake was further increased to six a day. So some people respond to dietary cholesterol with elevations in blood cholesterol, while others don't.[10]

For those susceptible people, or responders, more than a moderately high daily intake of cholesterol (that is, above 600 milligrams) will raise blood cholesterol levels and will probably increase their likelihood of developing heart disease or strokes. Eggs are one of the richest sources of cholesterol (one yolk = 250 milligrams); despite the presence of some lecithin, they are not anyone's best ally in the war against atherosclerosis.

But an egg or two occasionally in the context of a largely vegetarian diet, with an otherwise low cholesterol content, is not likely to be a significant liability. Surveys show that the lacto-vegetarian's intake of cholesterol usually runs about half that of the general population.[11,12] With the added egg or two, intake would still be in what is probably a safe range even for those who are the most susceptible to the effects of dietary cholesterol.

Although for most people the amount of cholesterol in the diet may not in and of itself make much difference (unless it's extremely high), the relatively low level in the vegetarian diet does—in this case as before—seem to mark or identify a way of eating that is, in a number of more significant respects, less likely than usual to contribute to atherosclerosis. For example, quite apart from the question of cholesterol, vegetarians tend to eat less total fat, and as we've seen, the level of total dietary fat and oils seems to have more of an impact on blood cholesterol levels and on one's susceptibility to atherosclerosis than does the level of dietary cholesterol itself.[8]

We could leave the subject there, except for one major problem. Most people involved in the transition to vegetarianism are not simply in need of preventing atherosclerosis. Like the vast majority of Americans today, they already have it (see Phase 1), and need an approach that can reverse the process. To do this most skillfully, we must understand not only where the cholesterol deposited in the arteries comes from, but how to get rid of it.

An often-overlooked physiological fact is that bile salts, the substances in bile that are used to emulsify fats during digestion, are made from cholesterol. Bile is produced in the liver and stored in the gallbladder until a fatty or oily meal is eaten. Then it is squirted out into the duodenum, where it is mixed with the food. From there on out, the bile salts will take one of two courses: they may be reabsorbed during their passage along the intestinal tract and return through blood vessels to the liver, or they can pass out with the feces. The difference is crucial; if the bile salts (read cholesterol) exit with the stool, there is a constant reduction in total body burden of cholesterol, blood levels of it drop, and the process of laying down atherosclerotic plaque ceases. With sufficient removal, that process may even begin to reverse itself. At that point, one can eat a little cholesterol without getting into trouble. It will be used constructively.

On the other hand, if most of the bile salts are reabsorbed from the intestinal tract, outflow is cut off (see figure on p. 193). Cholesterol builds up in the system, and the way is prepared for diseases such as gallstones and coronary artery obstruction to develop. It should obviously be of great interest to Americans, the majority of whom die of atherosclerotic diseases, to understand what can be done to encourage bile salts to leave with the stool rather than sticking around to clog up arteries. Research in the last few years has made it quite clear how that can be accomplished. The answer is fiber—not just any fiber, but the right kind of fiber, and in the right quantities.

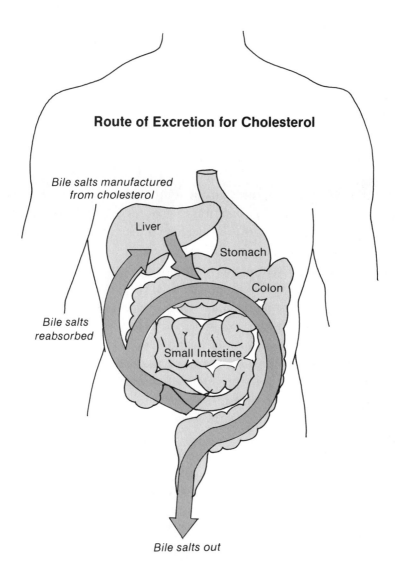

Route of Excretion for Cholesterol

Bile salts manufactured from cholesterol

Liver

Stomach

Colon

Bile salts reabsorbed

Small Intestine

Bile salts out

CLEANSING AND DIETARY FIBER

During the initial phases of eliminating various animal foods, one enjoys the benefits of a sort of cleansing. Meat, poultry, fish, cheese, and eggs are very rich, concentrated foods that are, without exception, devoid of fiber. The same is true, though to a somewhat lesser extent, of refined flour and sugar and of fats and oils. If such foods constitute a large proportion of what one eats, then the excretory functions of the digestive tract become increasingly inefficient. In the absence of the bulking effect of whole-vegetable foods, there is relative stagnation in the intestines. This can lead to difficulty in throwing out wastes as feces. Moreover, the flooding of the bloodstream with concentrated fats and protein, as well as the substances produced in the animal cells of meat, poultry, and fish during the deterioration that occurs after death, can all add up to produce a sort of molecular litter in the tissues. There are excessive concentrations of many useful substances, and the presence of others that are of no use.

This is an area where research scientists and seasoned clinicians often part company. Those health professionals who have worked for some time with nutrition and chronic disease frequently come to speak of wastes and deposits in the tissues that result from dietary excess. They may find themselves emphasizing the need for cleansing or "detoxification." Most laboratory scientists, on the other hand, find such ideas quaint and unscientific, since there is little in the way of research done from this perspective.

This is probably because our current methods and technology are not well suited to studying such matters. We can measure the presence of tiny amounts of any chosen substance in the tissues of the body—much as one could trace an identified man through a crowd. But we don't have the ability to step back and look at the internal molecular environment as a whole. We can say, in a sense, "The man we're trailing is *here,*" but we can't say, "The building is full of inappropriate, unnecessary, and irrelevant people who are in the way and are obstructing the normal orderly progress of business!" Yet it seems reasonable to assume that such a molecular clutter might develop in the cellular milieu of one who habitually takes in considerable quantities of unnecessary or unusable substances in his diet.

Though research is difficult and largely lacking in this area, there is a long tradition, both Oriental and Occidental, to support the notion that such conditions in the tissues contribute to the development of degenerative diseases. Atherosclerosis may be only one of the more obvious and easily detected versions of this process. It seems quite reasonable to postulate that in other chronic diseases, from arthritis to cancer, such a process might play an important role in impairing the body's inherent ability to resist breakdown and disorganization.

As one eliminates animal foods and begins to replace them with whole grains, legumes, vegetables, and fresh fruits, the situation is reversed. The bloodstream becomes less heavily laden with excesses, and the tissues are gradually able to mobilize and throw off their accumulation of wastes and deposits. The digestive system functions more smoothly and efficiently and there is a continuous and progressive process of removal of molecular clutter from the various tissues of the body. During the first months or even years after such a dietary change, one experiences an increasing sense of well-being, a growing lightness, a flexibility of limb, and a clarity of mind.

One's mental functioning and state of consciousness can be positively affected not only by the general systemic cleansing but also by the healthier condition of the gastrointestinal tract. Because of its myriad folds and rugae, the functional surface of the intestinal tract is immense, amounting to about 5,000 square yards. A healthy intestinal wall serves as an effective barrier, sealing off the contents of the gastrointestinal tract from the bloodstream. Chemicals from the environment and metabolic by-products of microbial growth cannot pass through such an intact wall.

But it does not seem unreasonable to postulate that inflammation and irritation from concentrated wastes, which are stagnant and undiluted for want of appropriate fiber, would compromise this barrier, allowing the circulation to be flooded with an assortment of miscellaneous substances that would disrupt metabolism and adversely affect normal physiological processes. Though the central nervous system is protected to some extent from such influences, it is not totally so, and mental and emotional processes could also be subverted, creating a sense of subjective clutter that corresponds to the molecular clutter in the bloodstream and tissues.

Cleansing, as conceptualized in the ancient systems of traditional medicine, referred both to the physical and the mental/emotional. The use of practical techniques for such cleansing often grew out of experience with intensive meditational introspection. The use of a wholesome vegetarian diet was one such technique, and it was highly regarded as an essential step in the direction of alertness and clarity of consciousness.

Clean, or Washed Out?

Such cleansing, however, is only one aspect of good nutrition. What begins as lightening and refreshing can, if continued too long, become depleting and weakening. Establishing a cleaner environment in the gastrointestinal tract and promoting the removal of wastes from the tissues may be important, but it does not guarantee adequate nourishment. A diet effective for cleansing may not be up to par in its nutritional content. Therefore it is important for one who intends to remain vegetarian for a long time to learn how to ensure and even, when necessary, bolster the nutritional content of a diet based on plant foods.

Perhaps this would not be a point of such critical importance were it not for the fact that the plant foods available currently in most of the industrialized world are of far less than ideal quality. Agricultural practices, based on the use of chemical fertilizers, on an indifference to soil erosion, and on a failure to encourage the growth of important microorganisms in the soil, have led to the production of plant foods that are often seriously deficient in vitamins, trace minerals, and protein.[13,14] (See also Phase 2, pp. 112, 133-34.) One who is conscious of this will, of course, use produce grown in healthy soils when available, but to the extent that this is not possible one must find other ways of increasing one's intake of protein, vitamins, and minerals.

Some might argue that the body will take what it needs and throw off what it doesn't, and that all that is necessary is to eat a larger quantity of fruits, vegetables, grains, and beans, and thus eventually enough nutrients will be extracted despite the quality of the food. Unfortunately, that is not a very practical solution, and the main reason it doesn't work is because of the presence of fiber.

Kinds of Fiber

There is much talk these days about the value of dietary fiber. An appreciation of its importance is long overdue. The typical American diet of animal products and refined foods has long been almost completely devoid of fiber; that recognition of this fact has been so slow to come is unfortunate. However, in the rush to dump quantities of fiber back into the diet, another equally obvious point has been overlooked: one can get too much. A person who tries to use bushels of anemic fruits, vegetables, grains, and beans to provide himself with the nutrients that he needs will find that eating a huge volume of such foods, all of which are high in fiber, leaves him feeling bloated and dissatisfied. Full of gassiness, he only confirms an English humorist's paraphrase of Shakespeare, "The vegetarian diet is full of sound and fury, but signifieth nothing." This problem is often further compounded by the tendency of misinformed zealots to lace nearly everything they cook with quantities of bran.

This is not to say that bran is never helpful. The typical American diet, being essentially fiberless, is probably less harmful after bran is added to it. There are many persons who will bear witness to improvements in health and bowel function after adding bran to an otherwise conventional diet. A good vegetarian diet, however, based on whole grains, legumes, vegetables, and fresh fruits, is already quite rich in fiber, and the addition of bran to such a diet is foolish, at best. Not only is the total content of fiber then excessive, but there is a disproportionate amount of certain types of fiber.

The word *fiber* has been used in the field of nutrition in various ways. Early attempts to measure the fiber content of a food involved exposing it to an acid and then to a strong alkali. The fibrous residue that wasn't dissolved away was called dietary fiber. This rather coarse material, predominant in the stems and peelings of vegetables and fruits and in the coverings of grains (bran), is high in cellulose. Cellulose is the basis of fibers like cotton, and is the major constituent of paper. But this is not the only indigestible part of plant foods. Besides this tough acid- and alkali-resistant material, which later came to be called "crude fiber," there were found to be other components of vegetable foods that the enzymes in the human intestine can't break down. Though they are grouped together with cellulose as total dietary fiber, these additional indigestible residues are not necessarily fibrous at all. They may even be gelatinous, as is the case with pectin.

Pectin is familiar as the thickener that is used to make jams and jellies. Like most of the other indigestible residue or fiber in the diet, it is complex carbohydrate—long, complicated chains of sugar molecules that differ from starch in that the linkages of the starch molecule are susceptible to the action of digestive enzymes, whereas these are not.

The indigestible fibers in plant foods such as cellulose come mostly from the plant's cell wall, which can be quite tough. By contrast, animal cells have only a delicate membrane surrounding them. This is all right because the structural strength of animals comes from their skeletal framework. Plants depend for their rigidity, however, on developing thickened cell walls. The collective strength of such cell walls is responsible for the plant's sturdiness.

There are basically two types of indigestible components that go into the construction of plant cell walls. The first of these, predominant during the early stages of the growth of the new shoots of a plant, are soft and tender. These materials are typified by pectin and are sometimes called "pectinaceous fiber." As mentioned before, they are fiber only in the sense of being indigestible. The second basic type of cell wall component is tougher and more rigid. This is added progressively as the plant cell gets older and is responsible for the toughness and strength of stems and hulls. The primary fiber of this type is cellulose. Its name means "cell sugar," since it is a chain of sugars and a major constituent of the mature cell wall. In fact, it is the most commonly occurring molecule in nature.

The sugar links of the cellulose chain are hooked together in such a way as to permit the chains to lie flat against one another. This results in a compact arrangement of fibrils that gives cellulose both its strength and flexibility. In larger plants, the cell wall may go on to become even woodier. This process is the result of adding an even stronger and more rigid component, lignin. Although lignin is prominent in the trunks and branches of trees and is the major constituent of wood, it is found in only small amounts in most plants considered edible. In fact, as a plant ages, and lignification proceeds, we are less and less likely to consider that plant appetizing. This is quite appropriate, since lignin is not only rigid, it is relatively impermeable to water, and so is unable to swell and provide the bulking effects of cellulose. Moreover, because of their rigidity, chunks of fiber that contain a significant proportion of lignin (stems, peelings, hulls) are more likely to be mechanically irritating to the delicate linings of the digestive tract.

Bran as a Source of Fiber

The same point can be made, though to a lesser degree, about plant material that is mostly cellulose with a smaller proportion of lignin. An example is the outermost covering of the grain, the pericarp, which is a major component of wheat bran. The fiber of bran is predominantly cellulose and lignin; only a small percentage of it is pectin. Unfortunately, until very recently our knowledge about fiber has been quite rudimentary, and a great deal was made of the nutritional value of bran before it was understood that most of its nutrients are unavailable. The protein in bran, for example, which will be at least 10% of its dry weight, is essentially indigestible because it is so closely bound up with cellulose.[15]

Though each kind of fiber has some beneficial properties, the gelatinous pectins would seem to be most soothing to the digestive system as well as the most effective in picking up and carrying out of the body the bile salts that serve as a mode of excretion for cholesterol. Lignin will pick up some chemicals that are cancer-causing, and cellulose will carry out others such as dyes[16,17] (see table below). But pectin is the critical fiber for the prevention or treatment of atherosclerosis.

An average American meat-based diet with added bran will supply cellulose and lignin, but no pectins to speak of. The cellulose is probably responsible for most of the effects for which bran is used. It absorbs water and is helpful as a bulking agent in a largely fiberless meat-based diet. Some of the cellulose is also broken down by bacteria in the colon to produce gaseous irritants. In small amounts these substances have a desirable laxative effect, but in excess they can cause severe irritation and pain.

Optimal Fiber Levels

Most available published information about the fiber content of foods is taken from early studies that tested only for crude fiber (cellulose and lignin), and reflect little about pectins and related residues. Thus, most figures for the fiber content of foods are virtually useless. A thorough analysis of the types of fiber in most common food plants has yet to be completed, and little has been done so far to explore the interactions between

Some Known Effects of Different Fiber Components

Fiber Type	Advantages	Disadvantages
Lignin	Binds some carcinogenic chemicals (e.g., nitrites)	Mechanically irritating
Cellulose	Binds other carcinogenic chemicals (e.g., dyes)	Binds some valuable minerals
Pectin	Binds bile acids	Binds some valuable minerals

Source: Inglett & Falkehag: *Dietary Fibers.*[15]

and among different types of fiber in foods. In other words, our knowledge about the intricacies of fiber in the diet is still in its childhood, if not its infancy.

Until more information is available, it seems safe to say that high-cellulose components of the diet, like bran, should be kept to a reasonable proportion of the diet. A vegetarian who eats large quantities of fresh fruits, vegetables, whole grains, and legumes will consume quite adequate amounts of such fiber. Not only should such a person find it unnecessary to add bran, he may even find it advisable to remove the woody, tough, and fibrous portions of vegetables and fruits in order to reduce somewhat his intake of cellulose and lignin. This means peeling many fruits, and peeling or even discarding the stems of certain vegetables, especially if they have grown to maturity and become tough. Such measures can appreciably reduce the tendency for a vegetarian diet to cause gas and bloating, by bringing its fiber content into a more optimal range.

Reducing the coarse-fiber content of the vegetarian diet also allows the body to more comfortably process a large quantity of nutrient-rich foods and extract more of the essential trace minerals, vitamins, and proteins. This is essential when we are dealing with plant foods that are grown on less than ideal soils, since such foods are likely to have lower concentrations of nutrients. Though a balanced intake of mixed fiber offers obvious benefits, a good vegetarian diet will supply enough, and it will usually be more useful to focus on concentrating the nutrients in foods rather than on increasing fiber, which would dilute those nutrients.

One approach to reducing fiber, concentrating nutrients, and working around the relative deficiency of minerals and protein in commonly available produce is to make fresh vegetable and fruit juices. This is best done with a juice extractor, which removes the nutrient-rich juice and throws aside the fiber. Most people would be slow to recover from the gassiness and bloating that would result if they tried to eat a pound of carrots between meals. But the glass of carrot juice that can be extracted from those carrots is quickly and comfortably absorbed, bringing with it a healthy dose of trace minerals and other essential nutrients.

MILK PRODUCTS: PROS AND CONS

Another way of adding protein, vitamins, and minerals without increasing the burden of dietary fiber is through the use of eggs and dairy products. When we use such foods we capitalize on the fact that nature has designed them to contain the highest possible concentration of nutrients for nurturing life. Milk and eggs are formulated in such a way as to be complete foods. That is, they can alone, without any supplementation, sustain life for protracted periods of time while the young animal has no other source of nourishment.

Research has shown, for example, that a lactating mother will secrete in her milk even minerals of which she has only very little. An old adage runs, "For every child, a tooth," in recognition of the fact that the mother will demineralize her own teeth and bones in order to keep the calcium levels of her milk high enough to sustain the growth and health of her child. We take advantage of this imponderable quality of motherhood when we rely on dairy products to bolster a diet from crops that tend to be deficient. Even though the grass, foliage, or fodder given the cow may also be less than rich in essential nutrients, the milk, we can be assured, will be of better quality. We rely on the cow to sift through, as it were, the vegetable matter, taking out and concentrating the more scarce but critical nutrients in her milk.

It is widely recognized that milk is a rich source of nutrients. Dr. Roger Williams, a highly respected nutritionist who discovered pantothenic acid, wrote that laboratory studies consistently support the idea that milk is an outstandingly well-rounded food for young or old and one that is difficult to match. "Almost any animal consuming a diet free from milk or milk products will have its condition improved if some milk is added."[18] Recent research promises to improve even further the image of milk as a dietary staple: dairy products have been reported to play a protective role in cancer,[19-21] perhaps by enhancing the immune response,[21] as well as to lower blood levels of cholesterol.[22]

The amino acid makeup of milk is excellent and can be used to supplement that of grains. While legumes do this even more efficiently, boosting the usable protein of grains more dramatically

A Sample Lactovegetarian Main Lunch and Light Supper

Lunch

> *garbanzo stew with rice*
> *spinach with paneer chunks*
> *green salad with yogurt dressing*
> *pita or chapati*

Supper

> *soup made of mushrooms and onions sautéed and*
> *blended with milk*
> *whole wheat toast*
> *fresh fruit with whipped paneer topping*

(see pp. 90-96), the amount of beans that some people are able to tolerate comfortably is limited. For this reason, many lacto-vegetarians find it convenient to organize one meal a day, usually the main meal, around the grain/legume combination and one lighter meal around a grain and dairy combination. (See above.)

Lactose Intolerance

Nevertheless, there are obvious and well-recognized disadvantages to the use of milk. There is no question that milk is not designed for consumption by adults. In fact, most people begin to lose their capacity to digest the carbohydrate in milk somewhere between the ages of eighteen months and four years. This is the result of a reduced production of the enzyme lactase, which breaks down lactose, the sugar in milk. Lactose that isn't broken down in the small intestine ends up in the colon, where bacteria there feast on it, producing gas and causing bloating, cramping, and often diarrhea.

Though a majority of adults in the world have a relative deficiency of lactase and experience such symptoms of lactose intolerance when they take large quantities of milk,[23] most would have to drink a quart at a time for that to happen. Only about 1 adult in 20 will have problems from the amount of lactose in an 8-ounce cup of milk. In fact, the usual level of lactase in adults is 5% to 10% of what it was in infancy, a time when the entire diet is milk and lactose accounts for the major source of energy. A decline in adulthood to 5% to 10% of the infant's level is quite an appropriate adaptation for a diet that may have only 5% to 10% of its calories as lactose from dairy products.

The persistence of lactase is more complete in those racial groups in which dairying has been common for many generations. Only 7% of the people of Switzerland, where pasturing cows form a traditional part of the scenic landscape, are lactose-intolerant, even with the large amounts of lactose that are present in a quart of milk, whereas 85% of Japanese (for whom a cow is a novelty) show such a response.

Black Americans are more likely than whites to be lactose-intolerant, but they may not be, depending on their ancestral origins. A study in Nigeria found that the incidence of lactose intolerance ranged from 99% in nondairying tribesmen to 20% in tribes wherein dairy herds were traditionally kept. Again, lower levels of lactose are probably well tolerated by the majority, and studies dating back decades ago showed an improvement in health and growth in most black children when milk was added to the diet.[24] Nevertheless, when marked intolerances do occur, and black children are forced to drink milk, medical and behavioral problems can ensue.[25]

Yogurt and Lactose-Reduced Milk

Fortunately, milk can be incorporated into the diet in ways that circumvent this problem. Yogurt is produced by a bacterial culture that breaks down lactose to lactic acid, producing yogurt's characteristic tartness. Though the percentage of the lactose actually broken down by the bacteria is small, bacterial lactase survives the stomach's acid and is active in the small intestine, where it supplements one's own (reduced) levels of the enzyme.

Thus, even those who are strongly lactose-intolerant can usually use a good-quality yogurt without difficulty.[26]

Yogurt is not only useful for those who are intolerant of lactose, it has long been credited with miraculous health-giving properties of its own. While many of these may be nonexistent and others exaggerated, it seems that current research is validating a surprising number of yogurt's reputed benefits. Although the point was long disputed, it now seems well accepted that yogurt can improve the microbial population of the intestine, providing a type of bacteria that may prevent the production of harmful substances, some of which could cause cancer.

Unfortunately the yogurt usually available in today's super-markets is not necessarily the same food of legend and fame. As with other foods that are fermented, the process can go awry. Many of the beneficial properties of yogurt derive from the type of bacteria growing in it. These can vary dramatically, and in many commercial yogurts the deciding factor in the choice of bacterial cultures is shelf life rather than health benefits.[nt.2] Some products sold as yogurt are merely milk with gelatin added. Similar problems are found with commercial cheeses, which are often contaminated with undesirable organisms such as molds, though cheeses do generally have the advantage of being well tolerated by those who have trouble with lactose,[27] probably because most of the lactose is lost during curdling and goes off with the whey.

Recently, lactose-reduced milk has been marketed that is produced by breaking lactose, which is a compound sugar, or disaccharide, into its constituent simple sugars (glucose and galactose). In contrast to fermentation, in which lactose is converted to lactic acid, lactose-reduced milk is not sour. In fact, its taste is even sweeter than ordinary milk, since both glucose and galactose are perceived as sweeter than lactose itself.

Dishes that incorporate milk into the recipe are also often well tolerated and are a part of traditional cooking in many areas where dairy products are an important source of nutrients but where a significant percentage of adults cannot handle large quantities of plain milk easily.

Milk Allergies

Milk allergy is a completely separate and distinct problem, and has nothing to do with lactose, though the two are often confused. Allergic reactions develop when the body pegs as foreign a certain protein and marshals its immunologic defenses against it. One can overreact to milk proteins in this way, but doing so is unusual unless there has been some overriding physiological or emotional reason.[nt.3]

The most common cause of milk allergy is giving cow's milk to infants in the first few months of life. The intestinal tract of the infant is immature and unable to filter out foreign substances well. Human breastmilk usually creates no problems, but cow's milk contains substances that are not appropriate to enter the bloodstream of the human infant, and against which antibodies are then made. This sensitizes the child, much as a vaccination would, and the child is thereafter "allergic to milk."

The use of milk products by a person who has become so sensitized can result in minor allergic reactions or more serious problems such as eczema or asthma. If at all possible, infants should be nursed until the age of four months to six months, and all other sources of nourishment avoided until at least the fifth month.[29,30]

Minimizing Milk Risks

Milk is also susceptible to many of the problems that affect other foods of animal origin. Toxic environmental chemicals such as PCBs and pesticide residues can show up in milk as they do in other animal foods. PCBs are not a common contaminant in milk, appearing primarily as a result of dairy cows eating silage from silos treated with the chemical. But pesticide residues have been of more concern, since they have been found in milk at levels even higher than those in meat and poultry. Fortunately the environmentally persistent insecticides have been discontinued and are fading from the food supply. Even mercury can contaminate milk, but levels in most areas run about a tenth of those found in fish.[31]

A more serious problem with milk is related to sanitation,

since milk is an ideal culture medium. That is, because of the nutrients it contains, it readily grows microbes. Warm milk is particularly susceptible to becoming spoiled by the growth of germs, so it is generally cooled as soon as possible after collection. But the skin of the cow, the milking machine (or hands of the milker), and the containers into which the milk is put are all sources of contamination. Moreover, certain bacteria or viruses can enter the milk from the cow's body. For such reasons the federal government has set regulations for the handling and treatment of milk. Pasteurization is required, and milk is checked periodically for levels of microbes.

Unfortunately, pasteurization is not a very thorough method of eliminating microorganisms from milk. It requires only that the milk be raised to 161° Fahrenheit for 15 seconds. Compared to boiling, which is 212°, this is not a very high temperature, and it is not expected that it will eliminate all microbes. Standards set for permissible levels allow counts up to 20,000 bacteria per milliliter (5 milliliters = 1 teaspoon) upon leaving the pasteurizer. In the 40° temperature of the typical refrigerator, the population of microorganisms doubles every 35 to 40 hours. The Consumers Union found that one out of six milk samples bought from retail grocers had counts over 130,000, with some running into the millions.[32] Interestingly, not all the contaminated samples were felt by tasters to have flavor defects.

The number of microbes is not the only issue; the type is also important. Dairy herds, unlike beef cattle, are not routinely fed small doses of antibiotics. But the cows do often receive routine doses of antibiotics for the treatment or prevention of such problems as mastitis, and milk, like meat, can contain antibiotic-resistant organisms such as salmonella.[33,34] Salmonella contamination has been especially common in dry milk, and such milk should be reconstituted and boiled or used in cooking.

To be safe, all milk should be boiled, including that which has been pasteurized. Though milk used in cooking will generally be heated sufficiently to sterilize it, it is especially important to boil milk that is to be drunk or used on cereal. After boiling it can be cooled, put in a clean container, and refrigerated.

Boiling will also destroy other microbes that could cause disease. Standard procedures for inspection do not check for many nonbacterial microorganisms, such as viruses. Multiple sclerosis, a disease that has been variously attributed to infection by slow viruses or by spirochetes, may be more common with increased milk consumption,[35,36] at least in countries where milk is not boiled before using.[36, nt.4]

Using Milk Skillfully

It is interesting to note that in India, a culture with long experience in using dairy products, it is routine to carefully boil all milk before use. Long ago researchers found that children given boiled milk showed improved health and growth compared with those on pasteurized milk.[37] The boiling is probably wise for other purposes in addition to those related to hygiene. For example, it may inactivate certain biologically active constituents of milk, such as hormones that could otherwise affect those who drink it.

Milk is a food that is designed to produce growth. This and other of its qualities are probably best understood in Ayurvedic medicine. In the Ayurvedic tradition the subtle properties of different milks—that of the cow, buffalo, goat, elephant, and even the camel—are well recognized and used therapeutically. In Ayurvedic terms milk is *kaphic,* that is, it is designed to produce substance and matter. Of all foods, it is the one that is probably the most intensely matter-producing, since it is designed to encourage growth in the infant. Matter that cannot be incorporated into the growing process, however, is of no use and must be gotten rid of. Thus is the case of milk taken by the adult who is not growing. The residue or waste (mucus) from this process is also referred to as *kaph,* and the origin of the English word "cough" is related to this Sanskrit root. Certainly the mucus-forming qualities of milk are one of its most widely recognized liabilities.

While the lactovegetarian cultures of the East are aware of the liabilities of milk products, they also have long experience in dairying, a profound appreciation of the value of milk, and an extensive repertoire of techniques for working around its liabilities. According to Ayurvedic precepts, milk is best taken in small to moderate amounts, and boiling improves its digestibility. Milk that is merely pasteurized is not so well handled, forming large lumps in the stomach. Although the chemistry of milk protein is very complex and its reaction to heat is not well understood,[38] it seems likely that pasteurization is sufficient to denature the large molecules of protein, disrupting their normal arrangement so they collapse and tangle, but that boiling breaks some of the molecules apart into shorter chains or even into individual amino acids, which can facilitate their absorption. According to tradition, when used in this way and in limited quantities, the mucus-producing tendency of milk is minimized. Cooking with milk—that is, adding it to vegetable dishes, for example, during the cooking process—not only exposes the milk to boiling temperatures, but also allows it to interact with the foods being cooked. It also ensures that the proportion of milk to other foods is appropriate. But from the perspective of Ayurveda, drinking quantities of cold milk alone is foolish and sure to produce excess mucus in the body.

Another widely used and very successful technique for incorporating milk products comfortably into the diet is through the preparation of homemade cottage cheese. This cheese is not prepared with rennet, as is the commercial product, but rather with lemon juice. This has the added benefit of imparting the beneficial nutrients of the lemon to the preparation (see recipe on p. 210). The effect of the acid upon the already boiled milk is not only to curdle it, but to further the hydrolysis of the protein, that is, its breakdown into constituent amino acids. This means that it is, to some extent, predigested. The curd or cheese is strained off and used as a key staple in many favorite dishes in the lactovegetarian cuisine of India. The liquid or whey is also highly nutritious and can be used for making breads or for drinking between meals as a cool, refreshing beverage that supplies a number of valuable minerals that are not kept in the curd. It is commonly believed among dairying peoples that it also provides the benefit of soothing and cleansing the urinary tract and reducing the tendency of the body to retain excessive water.

Fresh Cottage Cheese (Paneer)

The cottage cheese found in grocery stores usually contains additives and lacks freshness. Paneer, a homemade variety prepared in India with lemon juice, tastes fresher and better and also gives one access to the whey, a very healthful beverage.

To make about one cup of such cheese, simply bring one-half gallon of 2% milk to a foaming boil and add enough lemon juice to curdle it. Stir the milk and a bit of lemon juice together very briefly, wait a second, and then add more. Continue until the whey begins to look nearly clear. Allow the milk to boil for another few seconds. Then leave the pot undisturbed so the curd can separate from the whey. The liquid whey can be poured off while holding the mass of curd with a large spoon, or it can be strained through a thin cloth draped over a colander. Using a cheesecloth allows one to squeeze out enough whey to create a tighter "cheese" that can be cubed and will not fall apart when cooked in vegetable dishes.

*   *   *   *

Paneer can be used in a variety of ways:

1. Strain it dry, cube it, and add to cooking vegetables.

2. Use it in any recipe instead of cottage, ricotta, or cream cheese. Cheese cake, lasagna, and sandwich spreads, for example, are delicious when made with paneer. It can also replace soybean curd (tofu) in many recipes.

3. A rich and creamy dessert topping that is especially appealing on fruit salad can be made by whipping moist paneer in a blender with a bit of boiled milk. It can also be used to make a rich, high-protein, low-fat dressing for green salads.

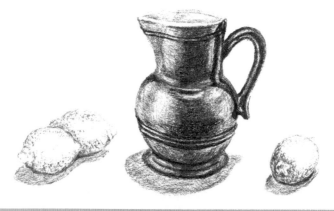

The cheese, called *paneer* in India, is probably one of the best-tolerated of the animal protein preparations and can be used in the diet on a daily basis. It does much to boost the protein content of dishes to which it is added, as well as providing additional food value without adding fiber, so as to avoid raising fiber content beyond the optimal range. Although paneer resembles tofu in appearance—both are white and often cubed before adding to vegetable dishes—they are not interchangeable. Though both are rich in protein, the amino acid makeup of paneer is better, it may be richer in some trace minerals, and it carries other benefits of dairy products, such as the B_{12} that tofu lacks. An ideal vegetarian diet might include both paneer on a daily basis and tofu several times a week.

Currently one of the greatest objections to milk is its butterfat content. Not only does the butterfat in milk contribute dramatically to total fat levels in the diet, but it contains significant amounts of cholesterol. For this reason some health experts recommend nonfat (skim) milk. Yet, in experiments, rats given nonfat dry milk developed atherosclerosis while those given milk with butterfat did not.[39] Moreover, since butterfat may play some beneficial role in the absorption of calcium,[39] and since dairy products are often an important source of dietary calcium, it is wisest perhaps to use lowfat (2%) milk. This reduces fat intake considerably (see diagram below), yet leaves enough to improve palatability and perhaps to assist with the absorption of calcium.

Percentage of Fat in Milk (by Calories)

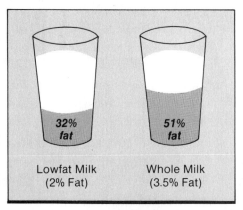

Lowfat Milk	Whole Milk
32% fat	51% fat
Lowfat Milk (2% Fat)	Whole Milk (3.5% Fat)

CHOOSING A COOKING MEDIUM: BUTTER VERSUS OIL

In almost every part of the world, food preparation involves the use of some fat or oil as a cooking medium. Generally what is used is to a large extent influenced by availability. Where pork is a staple in the diet, lard is common. In the Mediterranean area, where olive groves flourish, olive oil is favored. In dairying cultures, butterfat is used for most cooking purposes.

In North America, availability is less of an issue. Shoppers usually have a wide choice of cooking fats and oils, ranging from pure olive oil, and butter, to deodorized and bleached mixed vegetable oils or hydrogenated vegetable "shortenings" and margarines. Prices vary, but, in general, the vegetable oils and fats have become progressively more affordable, while butter has become more expensive. For this and other reasons, vegetable oils and vegetable fats have come to be used with increasing frequency. Liquid vegetable oils are used almost exclusively for frying and for salad dressings and mayonnaise, while solid vegetable shortenings are used for baking. Margarine frequently replaces butter at the table. Since the vegetarian may consider a shift to these plant products a logical part of the transition to vegetarianism, it is appropriate to look carefully at their effects.

Vegetable Oils in the American Diet

Vegetable fats and oils have always been a part of the diets of persons who consume plant foods, because all plants contain some fats and oils. But the use of extracted vegetable oils as a cooking medium or as a basis for condiments such as salad dressing and mayonnaise has been infrequent. In times past it was difficult, if not impossible, to extract oil from most sources, the most feasible sources being traditional ones such as olives and sesame seeds. Despite the winsome Madison Avenue-bred Indian maiden who holds a bottle of corn oil while confiding that her people always relied on "the golden goodness of maize," very little oil can be extracted from a kernel of corn with an American Indian mortar and pestle. The use of oils from plant sources such as corn had to await the advent of complex equipment.

After World War II the technology needed to extract oils from many grains and seeds became widely enough available that the oils became affordable and could compete with more established dietary fats like lard and butter. During the next three decades the consumption of vegetable oils rose approximately threefold.

In the 1950s it was noted that an increased intake of polyunsaturated oils lowered blood cholesterol. While some vegetable oils have only a small to moderate amount of polyunsaturated fatty acids, others such as safflower, corn, soy, and sunflower seed oils have a great deal. Since research was pointing to an association between elevated cholesterol levels and heart disease, it was suggested that increasing one's intake of these highly polyunsaturated vegetable oils might, by lowering blood cholesterol levels, cut one's risk of heart attacks. A number of large-scale experiments were done to test this possibility, both on healthy persons at risk for heart disease[40,41] and on persons who had previously suffered heart attacks.[42,43]

The results were initially encouraging. In one study in Los Angeles, deaths from heart disease were 70 out of 408 in the control group, compared with 48 out of 400 in the group on a diet high in polyunsaturates.[40] Two other trials showed more limited[41] and short-term[43] benefits, while another failed to show any improvement.[42, nt.5]

Even where the best results had been obtained, however, there was little if any reduction in total deaths.[44] Moreover, in the study that had shown the most encouraging results, that done in Los Angeles, there was an unexpected complication. After reviewing their results, the research team was moved to publish a paper pointing out that the incidence of cancer in the experimental group that had taken the polyunsaturates was nearly double that of the controls, who had not taken the increased levels of vegetable oils.[45] Though the other three experiments apparently did not result in more cancer, this finding was disturbing.[nt.6]

Polyunsaturated Oils and Free Radicals

Meanwhile, in the early 1960s another line of enquiry had started among oil chemists, who noted some properties of polyunsaturated oils that made them seem unsuitable for use in the diet. They began to publish these findings in their journals over the next decade.[47-51] Many of the effects seemed to stem from the marked tendency that polyunsaturates have for rancidity. When there are two unsaturated spots in the fat chain, oxygen will tend to pick off a hydrogen atom, forming a peroxide fragment, which is highly reactive, and leaving an unpaired electron where the hydrogen was (see figure on p. 215). That spot in turn also becomes very reactive. Until it combines with something, it is called a free radical. Each of these mischief-makers, the free radical and the peroxide fragment, is quick to react with other molecules that it contacts. This produces molecular damage and more free radicals. What results is a sort of chain reaction perpetuating these destructive particles and leaving in its wake a trail of useless molecules. When the peroxidation and free radical formation occurs within the body, cells can be damaged and may, as a result, behave abnormally or die.

Certainly polyunsaturated oils are not the only causes of free radical formation. The tissue damage resulting from radiation is based on the same mechanism, as are many other destructive effects on the body. It is thought that it is through lipid peroxidation that alcohol damages the liver.[53] Cigarette smoke produces free radicals by oxidizing polyunsaturated fatty acids in the body.[54] The toxicity of such environmental contaminants as mercury,[55] PCBs, dioxins, and pesticide residues are thought to involve free radical formation,[56] as is the carcinogenic action of aflatoxin.[57]

In fact, the effects of many, if not most, cancer-causing agents are thought to involve the formation of free radicals, which readily damage DNA.[58,59] It is the alteration of the DNA molecule, in which are encoded the instructions that govern the functioning of the cell, that is thought to be one of the major events that can set off a malignant process. The cell's normal functions are abandoned in favor of an unbridled reproduction, dictated by a distorted DNA code.

Polyunsaturated Oils and Free Radical Formation

Linoleic acid

· Free radical

Peroxy radical

Both the hydroxy radical and the peroxy radical will tend to pick off hydrogen atoms (-H) from additional linoleic acid molecules, forming two more free radicals. It is thus that such polyunsaturated oils, in the presence of atmospheric or tissue oxygen, trigger chain reactions of radical formation.

Source: Brisson: *Lipids in Human Nutrition.*[52] Halliwell & Gutleridge: *Free Radicals.*[57]

Oxidation is the basic process in free radical formation, and ozone (O_3) is another powerful initiator.[60] A high ozone count can cause an irritation in the lining of the respiratory tract that is based on free radical formation.

Controlling Free Radicals

Though free radical activity is capable of great destruction, it is not always undesirable. In fact it is through precisely this mechanism that the white blood cell is able to destroy the bacteria it engulfs. It merges the microbe with a pocket of free-radical-producing substances and thereby breaks it apart. The trick is to control the chain reaction. As long as such activity can be contained, it can be harnessed for constructive purposes in the body. Once it gets loose it's like wildfire, and will spread until the reactive substances are neutralized and the flames are quenched.

Certain enzymes and specialized molecular systems in the body are designed to inactivate free radicals. They serve to keep the reactivity of the process in bounds and to defuse rampaging radicals that have escaped their normal confines. Examples are superoxide dismutase, an enzyme that contains manganese or a combination of zinc and copper, and glutathione peroxidase, a selenium-dependent enzyme. Other free radical quenchers or scavengers are vitamin E, vitamin A, beta carotene, and probably vitamin C.

In the 1970s a number of reports emerged attributing to such antioxidants the ability to reduce the incidence of cancer.[61-63] Beta carotene, for example, had previously been thought to be valuable only as a raw material from which vitamin A is made. It turns out, however, that carotenes are synthesized in plants for the purpose of protecting them from the free radicals that are generated by the ultraviolet radiation of sunlight to which they are exposed during photosynthesis. As a result, carotenes have excellent antioxidant properties.[64] A recent study of elderly people showed that those taking the most carotene-containing foods had a risk of cancer that was less than a third of those who took the least of such foods.[65] Yellow vegetables contain substantial amounts of carotenes, but it is in the green leaves of vegetables where photosynthesis takes place that enormous quantities are found. The presence of such antioxidants in whole foods probably accounts for the fact that the intake of vegetable oils as part and parcel of a whole-plant food is associated with a decreased risk of free-radical-related diseases like cancer, whereas the intake of most of the commonly added, extracted oils from plant sources has the opposite effect.[66-68, nt.7]

Turning the Tide

As long as the diet is rich in the antioxidant vitamins and the trace minerals, such as selenium and zinc, that are needed to keep the relevant enzyme systems replenished, one should be able to handle a moderate load of free radicals. The trick here is to create only a moderate load. Obviously a little bit of radiation or a little bit of vegetable oil is not going to be fatal. If the burden of free radicals is not heavy, controlling them is feasible, but the balance will shift if the tissues are inundated with environmental toxins, ozone, residues from cigarette smoke and air pollution, and the by-products of low levels of radiation. Add to that an intake of polyunsaturated fatty acids that has nearly tripled in the last 75 years,[78] and you may be in trouble.

If all the scavengers and quenchers are occupied in deactivating free radicals that are initiated by toxins, pollutants, and unstable oils from the diet, then none are left to carry out the necessary work of containing and focusing the purposeful versions of such reactions. In such a case, the potentially constructive free radical reactions propagated in the body may begin to run rampant. It is just such a situation that is thought by some researchers to give rise to inflammatory diseases like arthritis or allergies.[79, 80]

What we are talking about here is a constant struggle between those factors that tend to produce free radicals in the body and those that can inactivate and control them. As long as we are well nourished with adequate intakes of trace minerals and vitamins, and our lifestyle is such that we dump only a reasonable burden of free radical formers into our bodies, we can manage nicely (moving toward the left in the diagram below), overcoming and controlling molecular damage and harnessing free radical activity to ensure good health. If, however, nutrition is inadequate, or the burden of the free radical initiators is too great, we may find ourselves moving instead toward tissue damage, chronic disease, and perhaps premature aging.

As it became clear that so many of the events in life that cause normal wear and tear on the body, such as background radiation or exposure to toxic substances,[77] involve free radical damage to cellular components, gerontologists began to formulate a theory of aging that is based on the cumulative damage suffered from free radical activity. Many threads of evidence have strengthened the case for this theory.

It has been shown that the pigment (lipofuscin) that causes age spots on the skin and increases in the tissues with age is composed of peroxidized cellular components, primarily the unsaturated fatty acids that are a major constituent of cell membranes.[81] It is also thought that the loss of elasticity in connective tissue and skin that occurs with progressing age is due to cumulative free radical damage to the collagen fibers.[82] Dermatologists have found a fourfold increase in premature wrinkling and aging of the skin in those with increased free radical exposure due to taking extra polyunsaturated oils in the diet.[83]

The Struggle Between Free Radical Initiators and Inactivators[nt.8]

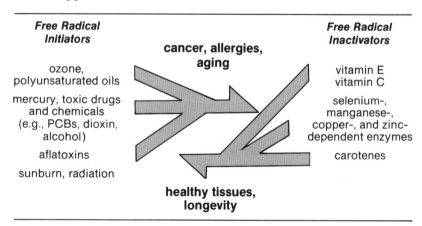

Free Radical Initiators	cancer, allergies, aging	Free Radical Inactivators
ozone, polyunsaturated oils		vitamin E vitamin C
mercury, toxic drugs and chemicals (e.g., PCBs, dioxin, alcohol)		selenium-, manganese-, copper-, and zinc-dependent enzymes
aflatoxins		carotenes
sunburn, radiation	healthy tissues, longevity	

What has come to be called the free radical theory of aging is further supported by evidence that some antioxidants and other free radical scavengers can extend the life span of experimental animals.[74,82] All this suggests that much of what we call aging may simply be the accumulation of damage that has occurred each time antioxidants and enzyme quenchers fail to control and focus free radical activity. According to this theory, aging would accelerate as control mechanisms are overwhelmed and free radical and peroxide levels rise. That this is so has been supported by measurements of lipid (fat) peroxide levels in the blood of different age groups: there was a gradually mounting level of peroxides, which increased each decade of life from childhood through age 70.[84]

A given organ is not affected by free radical damage to the same extent in every person. Such variations are attributed to the genetic makeup of the individual, which is thought to modulate the deleterious effects of free radical reactions in such a way as to create various patterns of deterioration. Those that develop slowly and that are nearly universal we call "normal aging," but if a pattern emerges earlier or is somewhat atypical, we single it out and consider it a disease. Such is thought to be the case with most of the degenerative diseases, including arthritis, diabetes, cancer, and also, perhaps, the atherosclerotic vascular diseases such as heart attacks and strokes.

Free Radicals and Atherosclerosis

The same lipofuscin that constitutes the pigment of age spots is also a major constituent of the plaques that clog the arteries affected by atherosclerosis.[47,81] This component is inert and indestructible and may lend a stubborn permanence to the deposits.[85] But free radical damage may play an even more primary role in the origin of atherosclerosis. While most of the attention in research on the disease has focused on the formation of the deposit, it is commonly accepted that plaques form in sites where there has been some prior damage to the endothelial lining of the artery. Japanese investigators showed that injections of the peroxides of linoleic acid (the most abundant fatty acid in the vegetable oils consumed by Americans) severely damaged the intima or inner lining of the aorta, the major artery leaving the heart. They concluded that an increased level of lipid peroxides in the blood can be the event that initiates the process of atherosclerosis. In keeping with this hypothesis, they found that both patients suffering from heart attacks and those who had strokes had levels of lipid peroxides in the blood that were double those of normal persons.[86]

Long before identifiable illness is produced, however, the adverse effects of peroxidation and free radical damage on vital organs such as the brain may interfere with one's functioning. Laboratory studies found that the number of errors made by rats attempting to navigate a maze increased as vegetable oil in the diet was increased. Learning ability suffered,[87] even though at the levels used there was no increase in mortality. This brings up the possibility that free radical damage could impair mental functioning without being severe enough to decrease life span. If the production of age pigment, so prevalent in the senile brain, is related to free radical damage, it is not surprising that we are seeing an increased population of elderly people who are still physically functional, but not mentally so.

Though serious reservations about the inclusion of poly-unsaturates in the diet may be more than justified, even when they are of the best quality, the fact is that much of the oil consumed today is damaged by deep frying. Fast-food outlets are notorious for what oil chemists call repeated-use frying. When oil is raised to the temperatures commonly used for deep frying, about 400° to 425°, the unsaturated fatty acids not only tend to undergo peroxidation, they also begin to join together, forming chains and cyclic compounds,[88] many of which are known to be toxic. After 40 hours of use in a restaurant the oil will be sufficiently deteriorated[89] to be considered unfit for consumption. In Europe restaurants are monitored and the use of such oils is prohibited, but in the U.S. it is the custom simply to add oil to deep fryers rather than periodically replacing it.

Margarine and Vegetable Shortening

One way to deal with the risks of polyunsaturated oils is to saturate them. This is done by bubbling hydrogen gas through the oil (in the presence of a catalyst such as nickel) so that the empty spots in the fat chain are filled with hydrogen. This produces a "hydrogenated vegetable fat." Examples are vegetable shortening and margarine. The melting point of the oil rises after this process, so what was previously a liquid at room temperature is now solid.

This makes a product that is more convenient to use. Peanut butters are often hydrogenated so they don't separate, and cheeses so they remain firm and don't ooze. Hydrogenation not only provides a product that is more convenient and appealing, it also reduces the tendency of the oil to pick up oxygen and undergo free radical transformation. It also allows the fat to stand up better to heating. Hydrogenated fats are less likely than oils to polymerize and to form toxic by-products. The only drawback to this solution is that some of the fatty acids produced during hydrogenation are different from those found in nature. The shapes of some of the molecules formed are odd and may not be well tolerated by the body.

When the oil is hydrogenated, not all the empty spots in all the fatty acids are filled. The process is not allowed to go that far: if it did, the product resulting would be too hard—suitable perhaps for making candles, but not cakes. So ordinarily oils are only partially hydrogenated. This raises their melting point somewhat, but leaves them still moderately soft. Stick margarines are more thoroughly hydrogenated than tub margarines, but in both cases the process is only partial.

The most serious problem that results from making these vegetable fats, as they are called, is with the fat chains that don't get hydrogenated. While they may retain their double bonds, the hydrogenation may jostle them about a bit, shifting the position of the bonds and the shape of the molecules. The new versions are called trans-fatty acids, while the ordinary types are referred to as cis-fatty acids. These reshaped fatty acids are different from the ones prevalent in a diet from natural sources. It is clear that in some important ways they are not processed metabolically in the same fashion as those they have replaced. This has led some experts to maintain that these fats should be considered food additives rather than foods until their safety is established.[90]

Though even in a natural diet small amounts of trans-fatty acids can occur, in North America since 1940, due to the growing popularity of hydrogenated fats like margarine and vegetable shortenings, intake has approximately tripled.[nt.9] When included in the diet at levels common today, trans-fatty acids are incorporated into cell membranes.[94] Such membanes function abnormally; the mitochondria, the little compartments within the cell where fuel is burned, swell and show lower rates of energy production when their membranes are altered in this fashion.[91,94] A higher incidence of cancer is associated with diets high in trans-fatty acids, according to some reports.[91, nt.10] It is thought that perhaps the disruption of the cell membrane allows carcinogens such as free radicals more access to sensitive cellular components, especially DNA. The same might apply to other potentially destructive agents that are ordinarily kept out of the cell,[nt.11] such as high concentrations of calcium (see Phase 2, p. 126).

Butter's Little-Recognized Virtues

The failure of vegetable shortening and margarine to solve the defects of vegetable oils is a powerful argument for falling back on natural, saturated fats as a cooking medium. Since animal fats such as lard will be considered inappropriate by most vegetarians, and naturally saturated vegetable fats like coconut oil have been associated with an increased risk of heart disease,[97] only butterfat remains as a reasonable option, and it becomes important to examine its effects carefully. Butterfat does increase cholesterol intake and does, like any other fat or oil, contribute to the total fat intake. But if cholesterol levels in the diet are in a moderate range and thus not of concern, and if total dietary fat is low, as it tends to be on a vegetarian diet, then what is the effect of using butter?

In the first place, it is largely saturated and is less prone than vegetable oils to form free radicals. Moreover, it may offer some unusual benefits. For example, one of its constituents is butyric acid, a unique short-chain fatty acid that has been credited with anticancer activity, antiviral effects, and even biochemical properties that may be helpful in the prevention or treatment of Alzheimer's disease.

Although butyric acid is also produced in small amounts when soluble fiber such as pectin is fermented in the colon, it is not found in fats or oils other than butter, since it is the fermentation of vegetable matter that takes place in the rumen of the cow that makes it available for incorporating into milk. In fact, it is the fatty acid that gives butter its characteristic odor and flavor. While the remaining carbon chains in butter and those of other dietary fats and oils are longer—for example, palmitic acid has 15 carbons—butyric acid has only 4 carbons in the chain. A 15-carbon chain will extend all the way through the lipid bilayer membrane that surrounds the cells and the subcellular organelles such as mitochondria (see figure below); but butyric acid only goes one-fourth the way through. When incorporated into the cell membrane, it appears to confer some unique properties. For example, it increases the human cell's production of the antiviral substance interferon by 25%[98] and it inhibits the reproduction of viruses in the cells of tissue cultures.[99]

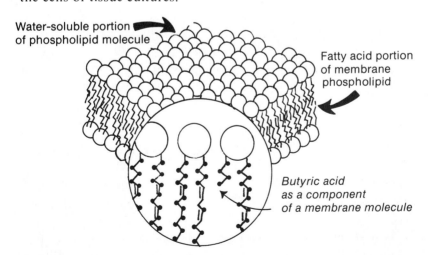

Water-soluble portion of phospholipid molecule

Fatty acid portion of membrane phospholipid

Butyric acid as a component of a membrane molecule

Butyric Acid in the Lipid Bilayer Membrane

Cells from malignant tumors in laboratory animals have been found to have less of a tendency to break away and travel to other parts of the body when treated with salts of butyric acid.[100] Malignant cells are more primitive or undifferentiated than normal ones, which is thought to be due in part to the fact that certain portions of the DNA molecule are not available to direct the cell to differentiate or mature. Salts of butyric acid (butyrates) seem to facilitate the unmasking of those portions of the DNA that are necessary for cellular differentiation.[101] In the presence of butyrates, malignant cells have become normal.[102] Since the same kind of interference with proper DNA activity that is involved in cancer is thought to play a role in aging, it has been suggested that butyric acid could provide a sort of anti-aging influence,[103] one that would complement the effects of antioxidants and free radical quenchers.

In view of such theories it is interesting to note that a common folk practice in India is to take a tablespoon of clarified butter (ghee) in the morning. Though modern nutritionists might take a dim view of such a habit, citing for example the cholesterol content of butterfat, those who have used it swear by it, insisting that it helps them maintain alertness and mental acuity as they grow older. Milk itself figures prominently in the regimens of Rasayana, a subdiscipline in Ayurveda devoted to rejuvenation. In view of this, it is intriguing to find that butyric acid has recently been credited with at least four distinct activities that might be of benefit in preventing or treating Alzheimer's disease.[103-9, nt.12]

Sometimes it almost seems that butter is assumed to be unhealthful because it tastes so good. But in view of what is known about free radicals and the pool of influences that tend toward degenerative disease, is it not conceivable that a craving for butter might be an appropriate if somewhat exaggerated response to the need to protect cells against malignant and infectious processes? Obviously, the solution to the problem of dangerous levels of destructive influences must include many changes in diet and lifestyle; nevertheless, a reasonable amount of butterfat might make a small yet significant contribution on the positive side. During the various treks he made around the world in the 1920s to study the relationship of dietary patterns and health, Weston Price was consistently impressed with the role of butterfat in promoting good health. His observations led him too to suggest that butter might increase longevity.[111]

Much of the negative feeling about butter comes from the fact that researchers have tended to lump it together with lard and beef fat. Because they all come from animals and all contain cholesterol, it has often been assumed that their effects are similar. But butter is different from other fats of animal origin in a number of ways. First and foremost, it is not a constituent of the animal carcass, as are lard and suet. It is, rather, a fat that is derived and produced specifically for nourishing, in the same way that milk itself is. One would expect that nature would provide it with special qualities for preserving and enhancing the quality of life. From this perspective, the suggestion that it might have unusual effects such as preventing viral infections, promoting healthy maturation of cells, or protecting the integrity of the nervous system do not seem far-fetched.

Another matter awaiting study is the difference between butter and ghee. In order to prevent the milk solids present in the butter from scorching and spoiling the taste of the food and to make it less perishable, butter is often clarified. This is accomplished by cooking it until its water content boils off and its milk solids settle out. (See recipe on p. 226.) The resulting product, clarified butter, or ghee, is a favored cooking medium in two of the world's greatest culinary traditions, French and Indian.

Classical French cooking relies heavily on clarified butter, and according to Ayurvedic teachings ghee has a preservative effect as well as a special capacity for picking up the medicinal benefits of seasonings and herbs and carrying them into the body. For this reason natural medicines made from herbs and spices are often produced in a ghee base that is thought to enhance their effect and to assure that they keep well.[112] It may be that the clarified butter protects foods and medicinal substances from deteriorating because of its resistance to oxidation. (The fatty acids of butterfat are relatively resistant to damage by oxygen, though its cholesterol content is another matter.[nt.13]) In any case, when food cooked in ghee is compared with that cooked in vegetable oils, after 24 hours of refrigeration there is often a noticeable difference in freshness and eye appeal.

Preparing Clarified Butter (Ghee)

Butter is not pure fat; it is also composed of water and of milk solids that are soluble in water. When the water is evaporated by boiling, these solids precipitate, and the oil or ghee remains.

To make ghee, heat unsalted butter in a saucepan until it boils; then lower the heat. When the white foam of milk solids that will accumulate on the top begins to collapse and thicken, start skimming it off. Do not disturb the bottom of the pan, as some of these solids will also sink and can be left in the pot until after the ghee is poured off. As the butter continues to boil, watch the oily portion to see when it becomes clear, and watch the sediment on the bottom to see when it becomes a golden brown. Don't let this scorch and ruin the ghee.

When all the water is evaporated, the sound of the cooking will change from one of boiling to one of frying, and the bubbling will stop. When only the clear, hissing oil and the golden sediment remain, the ghee is ready. At this point, the temperature will begin to rise quickly, so remove the pan from the heat, and let it sit for a moment. During this time, the hot fat will turn the sediment a little darker.

Pour the ghee off into an earthenware, glass, or metal container for use near the stove. Scrape out the sediments and refrigerate them with the skimmings, to add when cooking vegetables, sauces, or breads.

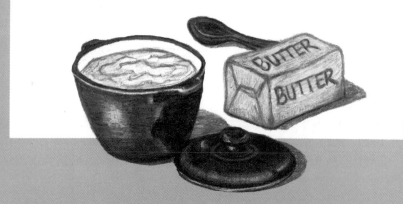

TRANSLATING PRINCIPLES INTO PRACTICE

Through the various sections of this book, as the issues relevant to sound vegetarian nutrition have been examined, one by one, the outlines of an ideal diet have gradually taken shape. It may be helpful here to pull together in one place the specifics of such a balanced, healthful, lactovegetarian diet, with concise guidelines for putting together commonly available foods to create it, and some hints on how to accomplish this within the confines of modern life, its time constraints, and its multiplicity of responsibilities.

Balancing the Vegetarian Diet

The balanced vegetarian diet has a few basic components that should be fairly consistently present, with other elements that are more optimal and that permit of considerable latitude. The most fundamental features of this diet are two: the grain/legume combination, and the cooked green vegetables. Next in importance, in the context of today's food supply, is the supplemental protein. The basic three elements might be represented as depicted on p. 228.

Grains may include rice, wheat, corn, oats, barley, millet, rye, and so on. Rice is, for many reasons, the most often preferred staple. Combined with a legume, it is nicely complemented by wheat (see Phase 2, p. 98). Although rice and wheat may be tolerated well on a regular basis, most people find daily repetition of the same legume to be tiresome. A variety of legumes is widely available, and each lends itself to a different and distinctive mode of preparation.

The third circle represents green vegetables. By this is meant fresh, cooked green vegetables. Salads or frozen vegetables will not fill the bill. Fresh, cooked string beans or broccoli or asparagus are adequate choices for occasional use, but the most ideal staples are the leafy vegetables. These include spinach, chard, kale, collards, mustard greens, turnip greens, beet tops, dandelion greens, escarole, vegetable amaranth, and others. Cabbage does not have the nutritional value that the darker greens have. Though

Basic Elements of a Vegetarian Diet

Supplemental protein/B_{12} source
10%

Vegetables
15-25%

Legume
10-20%

Whole grain
30-40%

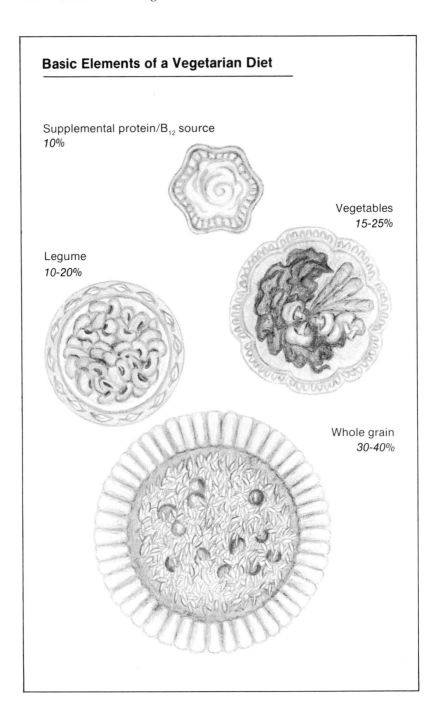

each of the leafy green vegetables is unique, as a group they tend to be high in protein, calcium, and carotenes. Each vegetable will be found to have certain strengths and certain weaknesses as a food. For this reason variety is desirable. This can be accomplished by using different vegetables on different days, or by preparing a mixed vegetable dish that includes several green and several nongreen vegetables.

In order to provide a dependable source of B_{12}, the supplemental protein should be from animal sources. Milk seems preferable for this purpose. Eggs can also be used, or if circumstances and preferences so dictate, fish can replace part or all of the milk and eggs. The quantity of this should be kept relatively small—perhaps sufficient to supply 5% to 10% of one's caloric intake. One example might be a half cup of cottage cheese, or a cup of yogurt. Soy protein such as tofu can be added occasionally (up to a half pound a day per person).

The diet should also contain some raw food at least once a day, preferably more often than that. (See figure on p. 230.) Fruits meet this requirement, as do green salads. Freshly squeezed or extracted juices, whether fruit or vegetable, also fall into this category, but should not totally replace the raw fruits and vegetables. A total daily intake of these raw foods might run as follows: a glass of freshly squeezed citrus juice in the morning; one piece of fresh fruit with breakfast; a (small to medium) green salad at lunch; a glass of vegetable juice (for example, fresh carrot and apple) in the late afternoon; one or two pieces of fresh fruit after supper.

Nuts and seeds can be a significant source of some nutrients, but should be used sparingly (see Phase 2, pp. 104-6). Since most nuts are borne by large trees, their nutrients are brought from the lower levels of the soil by deep root systems and may contain minerals missing from crops grown in depleted surface soils. Small quantities of nuts, cut up and cooked into rice, legume, or vegetable dishes, also add appeal and texture variation.

Seasonings and cooking fats account for a small percentage of the food, but have powerful effects. Herbs and spices should be used cautiously. Many of them are medicinal and some have been identified as containing toxic compounds such as free radical

The Balanced Vegetarian Diet

Food Category	Percentage of Total Calories
Grains (e.g., rice *and* wheat)	30-40%
Legumes (a variety)	10-20%
Vegetables (especially green and preferably leafy)	15-25%
Also onions, mushrooms, tomatoes, peppers, carrots, etc.	2-5%
Supplemental protein: milk and soy (and eggs or fish)	10%
Fruits and/or raw vegetables	10-20%
Nuts and seeds	2-5%
Juices	10%
Seasonings	1%
Cooking fat (butterfat)	0-10%

Translates into
Sample Menus That Incorporate Major Elements of the Balanced Vegetarian Diet

Rice and beans plus cooked green vegetable with paneer

Bean burgers on bun with side dish of green vegetable (e.g., steamed broccoli)

Pasta with bean balls and cooked green vegetable plus green salad

Bean enchiladas with cheese and green peppers

Note: Many menus don't incorporate green leafy vegetables easily. Many also require excess fat to make them palatable and may, in addition, lean too heavily on dairy and employ legumes too little.

initiators.[113-14] The safest are turmeric, cumin, and coriander in a ratio of 1:2:3. One should start with a small amount and roast them until golden brown in a bit of clarified butter.

Cooking: How to Get It Done and How Long It Will Keep

Although the sort of diet just outlined may be ideal, you aren't likely to find it in your local restaurant or in the frozen dinner

---

A typical day's menu might look like this:

morning: 8 oz. orange juice. Wait half an hour. Then:

1/2 cantaloupe or papaya

3 oz. dry cereal (whole-grain cornflakes) with, for example, banana, pear, strawberries, or blueberries

1/2 cup milk (boiled and cooled)

noon: 2/3 cup rice

1/4 cup cooked beans such as mung, pinto, lentils, etc.

2/3 cup cooked green vegetable such as spinach, kale, broccoli, string beans, etc., with 2 or 3 one-inch cubes of paneer

1 whole-wheat pita toasted and lightly buttered, or 1 piece whole-wheat toast

a green salad with yogurt or paneer dressing

afternoon: 8 oz. fresh juice, e.g., carrot-apple

evening: 8 oz. spinach soup made with milk, onions, mushrooms, carrots, and spinach blenderized together

1 piece lightly buttered whole-grain toast

1 cup of fresh, diced fruit, e.g., pear and honeydew, with a whipped paneer topping

The main meal may be moved to the evening, with the light meal taken at noon.

section of the supermarket, so a considerable degree of commitment to food preparation is necessary, as well as a willingness to struggle resolutely with the momentum of old habits. Since many people can devote only limited time to food preparation, cooking should be scheduled carefully. Each of the components of a balanced diet—the vegetable dish, the rice, and the beans—takes time to prepare. The beans and vegetable dishes are especially time-consuming. For this reason it helps to be able to cook enough for more than one day. Cooked beans (dahl) can be kept for three days. That means a single cooking of beans can be eaten on four successive days. "Some like it in the pot nine days old," according to the old nursery rhyme, but that, as one might guess, is a bit of an exaggeration. As a rule of thumb three days is reasonable. Vegetables are more fragile and don't store as well after they're cooked, so usually a cooked vegetable dish can be kept and eaten the next day, but after that it should be thrown out. Grain dishes will usually keep the longest. Rice will remain good for four or five days in the refrigerator if kept properly covered. (See chart below.)

But sometimes these rules don't hold: one may find that after two days a bean dish looks unappealing, tastes dead, and leaves one feeling heavy and unpleasant. It hasn't kept well. Why? There are a number of possible reasons. First, the ability of food to

Storage Life of Basic Vegetarian Staples

Food	Storage life
Vegetables:	
mixed summer	48 hours
kale	72 hours
Rice	4-5 days
Beans	3-4 days
Boiled milk	6-7 days
Paneer	4-5 days
Whey	2-3 days

withstand storage depends in part on how it is cooked. Without seasonings, it won't keep as long, since many of the seasonings act as preservatives. If one studies the history of herbs and spices, one will find that this was originally one of their major functions. It's now known that some spices act as antioxidants, while others retard bacterial growth. Sausage, for example, is pork mixed with sage; sage is a preservative. This principle was crucial in the days before refrigeration and freezing were available. Ground-up meats were mixed with different spices and seasonings to help prevent their spoilage. Salt and smoking were also used as preservatives, as has been ghee (clarified butter).

The next factor that influences the storage life of food is the refrigerator: in many households it is a disaster, and constitutes a major health hazard. If the refrigerator contains meat or poultry, the risk of contamination with antibiotic-resistant microorganisms is particularly high. Dairy products pose a lesser risk, but milk should be kept tightly capped until it is boiled, cooled, and put in a clean container.

Even without the serious hazards posed by contaminated animal foods, the family refrigerator is often a problem because outdated and spoiling foods are not removed. When food is decomposing, something is growing in it. Usually it's bacteria or molds, and often it's a conglomerate of many varieties of both. The refrigerator provides a dark, moist environment that can encourage such growth. Hence it's very important, if cooked food is going to be kept as a regular practice, to make sure that the refrigerator is scrupulously clean. Anything that looks at all strange should be consigned to the garbage can immediately, not left for another few days to see how it comes along. Though it may seem mundane or even humorous, this is a critically important issue. From the point of view of simple hygiene and common sense, it seems possible that certain of the diseases prevalent today are due in part to microorganisms propagated in refrigerators as a matter of course. Epidemiologists have found, for example, that cancer of the esophagus is significantly higher in those who regularly eat moldy foods.[115] In any case, food that is decomposing is tamasic, and even without a knowledge of specific toxicities we can be assured that its overall effects are less than desirable.

The condition of the containers in which food is stored makes a difference, too.[nt.14] If they are clean and tightly closed, if the food was boiled in the pot, if something very clean was used to transfer the food into the container, and if nobody has taken a spoon off the counter where everyone's dirty hands were and put it in the pot, then the food will keep well.

Another important factor is the consistency of the temperature of the refrigerator. If the refrigerator is kept at a constant temperature, the food keeps longer. When it is left open, or when warm food is put in it, the temperature of the entire contents of the refrigerator goes up and foods spoil more quickly.

Food that is dry will stay fresh longer than food that is wet. This doesn't mean that everything should be cooked until it's dry. But it's helpful to understand that a dish that's on the dry side will keep for a greater length of time, while something that's very wet and soupy won't keep quite as well.

With some attention to the conditions under which food is stored, one can set up a schedule, cooking beans on one day and rice on another, with vegetables being prepared on alternate days. This can make life much less hectic. But some foods will last longer than others just by their nature. As rice lasts longer than beans, and beans last longer than vegetables, vegetables also vary. Kale, cooked well with turmeric, cumin, coriander, and ghee, if properly stored, may last long enough to be used on a third day. But sliced zucchini, simply steamed and put in the refrigerator, won't look very appealing even a few hours later. That particular vegetable is simply more fragile. Vegetables like string beans, collards, and kale will keep longer than others. Combining the selection of vegetables with proper cooking, the use of herbs, seasonings, spices, and clarified butter, along with good hygiene and refrigeration, one can keep food safely for reasonable periods of time: beans can be used on three separate days, and vegetables at least the second day. If rice can be cooked twice a week, beans twice a week, and vegetables three times a week, cooking at home becomes a feasible goal. (See plan on p. 235.)

Shopping is also a time-consuming chore and one needs to

A Weekly Cooking Schedule

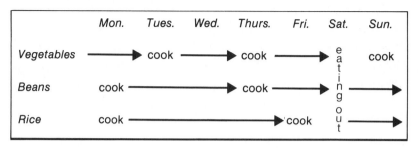

understand how long fresh, uncooked green leafy vegetables, for example, will keep. Of course, this depends in part on when they were picked, but it also has to do with how they are stored at home. The best way to keep produce is to sprinkle it with a little water, wrap it in a paper towel, and put it inside a plastic bag that can be sealed. That keeps the moisture inside, and green vegetables can be kept a lot longer that way.

Incidentally, spinach that is slimy-looking on its edges should not be used because it can form nitrites that are toxic.[4, nt.15] Most of the other green leafy vegetables are considerably more durable, such as collards and kale.

Keeping a kitchen stocked with fresh fruits that are ripe and appetizing can be an even greater challenge, though it's somewhat easier when one learns to use seasonal fruits that are plentiful. This may mean learning new uses for familiar fruits or learning to use fruits that are unfamiliar. Grains and beans are easier to come by. They can be bought in bulk and their variety is especially welcome in midwinter. This is a time to experiment with dried fruit and nut dishes and sprout salads. From the Balkans, for example, come recipes for beans cooked with dried fruit. Russia, with its nearly endless winters, has also done wonders with root vegetables and has given us borsht with black bread.

Different ethnic traditions have developed ways of preparing local vegetables that capitalize on their unique features, and we can learn from trying them. But meticulously following recipes is not generally a rewarding way to approach food preparation. What should be taken from ethnic recipes is their essence—the appreciation for the subtleties of the local foods and how to use them that has been evolved by trial and error over long periods of time. The most satisfying food is produced by a cook who assembles the best of what is at hand and then, on the basis of his or her appreciation of the principles of cooking and knowledge of different traditional dishes, combines those ingredients into a meal that is not only unique but fresh, vibrant, and wholesome.

Proceeding in this fashion, one can bring one's creativity to bear, and the preparation of food becomes a challenge that is both absorbing and enjoyable. One's attitude toward the preparation of food should reflect a general approach to diet that is based on flexibility and a willingness to explore and learn. Genuine (and lasting) dietary transition requires a constant observation of effects and an openness to change.

Maintaining such an attitude toward food and the nourishment on which life itself depends will allow one to gradually extend that attitude to other aspects of one's existence. Each daily experience with cooking or with eating then becomes an added impetus to regard life as a process of refining and evolving oneself.

If working with one's diet and with food preparation can be seen as a matter of self-discovery and self-transformation, then attention to diet and to cooking can be elevated from the realm of self-denial and of menial drudgery to become fascinating and fun. This just might be the single most important shift one can make during this transitional effort.

Using diet as a means to move toward greater clarity and awareness can only increase one's access to the physiological and psychological cues that will indicate which dietary changes have been of benefit and should be continued. From what we have learned in this book, if one continues to work consistently in this fashion, a gradual transition toward a healthful vegetarian diet would seem to follow naturally.

THE VEGETARIAN DIET IN PERSPECTIVE

AN OVERVIEW

In the course of this book we have looked in detail at a large number of controversial issues and in each case drawn some conclusions, many of which are at variance with what is commonly thought to be true. While each individual question is so interesting in its own right that it is easy to get lost in its intricacies, of most importance is how each of these points contributes to a comprehensive pattern. Therefore it might be helpful as the book draws to a close to step back and see how these various conclusions fall together to form an overall view of the relevance of vegetarianism today.

The Need for Change

First of all, it is clear that there is an urgent need for dietary change. The data cataloged in this book that reveal the relationship between diet and health are collectively overwhelming. There is very convincing evidence that one's risk of cancer and atherosclerosis, the two major causes of death and disability in our society, is dramatically reduced by the change from a meat and poultry diet to a vegetarian diet. A number of other common and troublesome disorders such as diabetes, high blood pressure,

237

osteoporosis, and obesity are also probably prevented or improved by a transition to vegetarianism. There is, in addition, some reason to believe that a vegetarian diet might contribute to longevity as well as have beneficial effects on psychological and emotional functioning.

The obstacles to making such an improvement in diet are not insurmountable. With only a little understanding it is possible to provide a vegetarian diet that is nutritionally sound or even superior, and at considerably less cost both to the individual and to society. The potential of a well-designed vegetarian diet to reduce or prevent suffering and disability is immense. In view of this, one might argue that the transition to vegetarianism is not a matter of mere taste or prejudice, it is almost a health imperative.

Though the evidence in favor of a vegetarian diet is compelling, experts still debate the advisability of altering the diet, expressing concern that more should be known about the effects of such change before it is adopted on a large scale. It is true that to mechanically recommend changes in eating habits as a response to correlations noted between dietary components and a specific disease creates the risk of causing other, perhaps more serious, problems. Such was the case, for example, when on the basis of an observed relationship between the ratio of polyunsaturated oils to saturated fats (the P/S ratio) on the one hand and heart disease on the other it was suggested that extra polyunsaturated oil be added to what is already one of the greasiest diets in the world. This does not mean that dietary change should be avoided, but that it should be tempered by common sense.

As we have seen, in this case the P/S ratio can be more appropriately lowered by decreasing meat and increasing vegetable foods. This introduces more polyunsaturates into the diet but not as isolated oils that are vulnerable to peroxidation and free radical formation. It also decreases total fat into the bargain. Why was such an obvious solution overlooked? Certainly in view of the facts, dropping meat and poultry from the diet appeals strongly to common sense. The persistence with which such foods are consumed, in view of the hazards currently associated with them and the many advantages associated with the vegetarian alternative, is difficult to understand. From such a perspective, it becomes increasingly evident that the consumption of meat is based not on reason, but on habit and inertia—or perhaps in some cases, on emotional factors.

How Did We Get Here, Anyway?

How could it be that we would find ourselves with such established and ingrained habits that are so thoroughly counter-productive? To find the answer to this question, we must try to see the present situation in its historical context.

Over decades and centuries the environment changes, eco-logical balances shift, and what is practical and expedient in one age may be inappropriate and anachronistic in another. Crowding and pollution are among the most prominent of the developments that have changed the face of the earth in the last century. Their influence has created conditions unsuited to the producing of healthful meat and poultry. Fish has also been affected to some extent, as has milk; even these animal foods, though somewhat safer, must be handled knowledgeably in order to use them to advantage.

So animal foods have become increasingly hazardous as well as decreasingly feasible economically. Attempting to feed the world with a meat-based diet is, in the final analysis, both foolish and impractical. Yet humankind has clung stubbornly to a pat-tern of meat consumption that should have been discarded and recognized as obsolete long ago. It is a pattern that was developed logically during an era of hunting but was perpetuated, perhaps unwisely even then, into a time when life and economics revolved around the small farm. To have carried it on beyond that, into industrial and postindustrial ages of urban living, was a mistake of considerable magnitude.

At this point in time, the consumption of meat seems to have become a sort of article of faith. The meat industry buys advertising time to portray beef as "real food." Their fingers unerringly on the public pulse, the admen sense that meat is a familiar constant for masses of people confused about what has nutritional value and what doesn't. Meat is an anchor in the tempest-tossed seas of a consumerism shaped by the conflicting messages of countless commercial interests. Through the morass of advertising, the consumer senses that most of the foods that are being promoted and that he or she is regularly consuming are overrefined, nutritionally depleted, and of little worth.

Though the mention of meat may still call up some confidence and vestiges of a sense of security, it anchors a nutritional vessel that is battered and worn and that is listing badly. Most of the foods that constitute the current diet are imitations, mere ghosts of the genuine items they have replaced. But meat, the anchor of this rickety ship, is itself also corroded and no longer reliable, for the quality of meat and poultry have declined along with the overall quality of the diet. So although meat remains in the diet, its complement of vegetables and grains has been replaced by increasing amounts of refined and processed starches, sugars, and oils, and meat itself has even less capacity than before to make up for what these supporting elements now lack.

Avoiding Extremes

An educated and well-informed public that has convincing data available will not long ignore it. It is becoming apparent that the benefits of vegetarianism for health and economics hold great promise, and dietary patterns have already begun to shift as a result. But it is most desirable at this point to make sure that new patterns about to be established are really optimal and don't constitute movements off onto tangents or extremes that carry risks of their own.

To respond to the massive amount of new data indicting animal foods by ceasing totally to use any of them may constitute such a risk. Certainly only a minute fraction of the world's vegetarians have traditionally followed a strictly vegan diet. A basically vegetarian diet supplemented with small amounts of animal food of the best quality available is much more common. Regearing dietary habits is expensive in terms of both time and effort. Adopting a diet that is unlikely to prove satisfactory is not only a huge waste, it is an experience that may discourage one and serve only to deter him from further attempts to make improvements in how he eats.

A Dietary Spectrum

Although a number of reasonable possibilities exist for those considering a new diet, the lactovegetarian diet seems destined to emerge as the most logical choice because it incorporates major improvements without taking them to extremes. The conventional North American meat-based diet of the mid-to-late twentieth century, and the strict vegan meatless diet, stand at either end of a continuum that encompasses much of the range of dietary habits today (see figure below).

The meat-based diet is high in protein, fat, salt, phosphorus, and calories, but quite low in fiber. It is more often accompanied by tobacco, alcohol, coffee, and sugar, as well as a host of chemical additives that are prevalent in the foods that currently make up such a diet.[4]

The vegan diet is low in protein, sometimes lower than is reassuring. It is low in phosphorus, too, which is an advantage, but

Nutrient Intakes of Lactovegetarians Compared with Meat-Eaters and Vegans

Midrange tends to correspond to optimal intakes; to either side one is likely to encounter excesses or deficiencies.

	Meat-Eaters	Lactovegetarians	Vegans
protein	85 g	55 g	35 g
fiber	4.5 g	8 g	15 g
salt	2.5 g	1.2 g	0.25 g
calories	2000 cals	1800 cals	1600 cals
calcium	1100 mg	900 mg	500 mg
phosphorus	1400 mg	1300 mg	800 mg

Sources: Freeland-Graves et al: *Zinc Status of Vegetarians.*[1] Abdulla et al: *Nutrient Intake and Health Status.*[2] U.S. Dept. of Agriculture: *Nutrient Intakes.*[3]

it is also low in calcium. It's rich in fiber—maybe even too much so. And it may be totally devoid of vitamin B_{12} and vitamin D.

The lactovegetarian diet is situated comfortably between these two extremes. Protein intake is probably optimal. Fiber is present, but not in such quantities that it will tie up minerals or burden the digestive tract. Vitamins B_{12} and D are adequate and reliably present. And it should be noted that the figures represented in this comparison derive from surveys of the diets of current North American lactovegetarians—diets that could without question be improved.

As a matter of fact, current American approaches to lactovegetarianism are varied and inconsistent. They are the result of a pastiche of miscellaneous influences: the return-to-nature values of the 1960s counterculture, remnants of the supplement-oriented health food movement that antedated the sixties, smatterings of various ethnic cuisines, and varying quantities of often contradictory scientific information. What emerges out of this melting pot is at best unpredictable. It's likely to involve clever, though not always nutritionally sound, imitation of favorite meat dishes, and to rely heavily on cheeses, eggs, and other foods high in fats and oils. Peanut butter and granola are ubiquitous. The use of legumes is, more often than not, rudimentary or absent.

The improvements that are needed in such lactovegetarian diets, and that have been indicated one by one throughout the course of this book, can upgrade their quality and begin to give shape to a way of eating that will provide a reasonable (and perhaps even optimal) goal for dietary change.

A Golden Mean

The diet that results will be, in a sense, streamlined. It provides for an efficient, uncluttered metabolism and avoids the pitfalls both of excess and of deficiency. A cleanly functioning body facilitates alertness of mind. Although such a diet embodies the principle of "less is more," it's well to remember that too little is still not enough. A regimen that is overly strict in some area—for example, the omission of all animal products—can create problems that are almost mirror images of those created by a diet that is excessive. The optimal diet is based on optima, not minima.

It's often felt that the vegetarian diet allows a smaller margin of safety than a diet based on meat, but this is not true if milk products are included. A movement away from the lactovegetarian range, either into a meat diet to the left or vegan diet on the right, will provide excesses of some nutrients, but insufficiencies of others.

Even a lactovegetarian does run certain risks: insufficient protein or B_{12}, for example, if a person fails to balance his diet properly. It may be true that a person on a conventional diet, in these respects, faces less uncertainty. He can be pretty sure he'll get enough protein and B_{12}. But he can also be relatively certain that he will have developed substantial atherosclerosis by the age of 50, and that he will by that time also face a high probability of cancer.

The risks that the lactovegetarian faces can be easily eliminated by following the practical pointers on how to plan and execute a well-balanced vegetarian diet that have been provided in the last chapter.

Vegetarianism and Consciousness

The transition to vegetarianism entails not only a leap forward in health, but a transformation of consciousness as well. While its effects on health are beginning to be widely acknowledged, its effects on consciousness may be slower to be recognized.

We have all adjusted to living with a diet that takes its toll on our well-being by presenting multiple challenges; some of these are deficiencies, some are excesses, and some are toxic substances. There is little doubt that we can cope with mild to moderate lacks of essential nutrients, various degrees of dietary excess, and rather massive onslaughts of toxic insults, such as free radical initiators. If this were not true, a large percentage of the population would not have survived this long.

But it is equally true that coping with toxins and deficiencies requires effort and energy. The resources expended in this way are not available for other purposes, such as creativity, self-development, and the exploration of the inner world. We might say that under such circumstances a person's attention is, to some extent, preempted by the necessity of coping with threats to his health and well-being. A portion of his consciousness is forcibly restricted to what are basically survival issues. A preoccupation with survival is the antithesis of playfulness and creativity, of selflessness and joy.

Eating in a way that is intrinsically self-destructive creates a split. It requires that a person constantly struggle to deal with the consequences of his own eating habits. Thus he pits himself against himself. Like any other conflict that operates within the mind, this bleeds off energy. It is the equivalent of an emotional complex.

For us to progress to a new stage of development we must carefully examine our way of living and divest ourselves of those habits that are most limiting. Especially important are habits that deplete our energy and that create problems that we must spend our potentially productive years struggling with. Those habits that perpetuate preoccupation with fear and survival are especially crippling and must be rejected if we are to progress to a consciousness that is constructive, cooperative, and less inclined to exploitation, hoarding, and suffering.

The transformation of consciousness is a complex matter. But if it can be furthered, even modestly, by simple changes in diet that yield many other benefits as a by-product, that seems a reasonable and appealing place to start. Its benefits for psychological and emotional life militate persuasively in favor of the transition to vegetarianism and will not escape the attention of those more thoughtfully attuned to changes within themselves.

Human evolution is built stepwise on small but significant changes in habits that bit by bit liberate consciousness from its confines. High-flown philosophies are of no use without practical change. Diet is one of the more practical aspects of life and one that is most accessible to change. Improvements in diet offer great potential both for the health of humankind and for the development of our individual and collective consciousness.

In fact, it may be no exaggeration to say that the transition to vegetarianism constitutes a critical step in the evolutionary process. Many forces conducive to this step seem to be converging at present. Whether it is taken now or whether it is taken later, its value becomes increasingly obvious and it would appear more and more as though the transition to vegetarianism is an evolutionary step that is inevitable.

NOTES

Commentarial notes, which are indicated in the text with "nt." preceding the note number, are listed for each chapter after the citational notes.

Why Vegetarian . . . and How

Citational Notes

1. U.S. Department of Agriculture, Economic Research Service: *National and State Livestock-Feed Relationships.* Statistical Bulletin no. 446, p. 76, Feb 1970.

2. Pimentel D, Oltenacu PA, Nesheim MC, et al: The potential for grass-fed livestock: Resource constraints. *Science* 207:843, 1980.

3. Lappé FM: *Diet for a Small Planet.* New York, Ballantine, 1971, p. xiii.

4. Szekely EB (trans): *The Essene Gospel of Peace.* San Diego, Academy of Creative Living, 1971, pp. 44ff.

5. Hopkins EW (ed): *The Ordinances of Manu,* 2nd ed. New Delhi, Oriental Books Reprint Corp., 1971.

6. Hardinge MG, Stare FJ: Nutritional studies of vegetarians, I: Nutritional, physical, and laboratory studies. *J Clin Nutr* 2, no. 2:73-82, 1954.

7. Hardinge MG, Stare, FJ: Nutritional studies of vegetarians, II: Dietary and serum levels of cholesterol. *J Clin Nutr* 2:83-88, 1954.

8. Hardinge MG, Stare FJ, Chambers AC, Crooks H: Nutritional studies of vegetarians, III: Dietary levels of fiber. *Am J Clin Nutr* 6, no. 5:523-25, 1958.

9. Register UD, Sonnenberg LM: The vegetarian diet. *J Am Dietetic Assn* 62:253-61, 1973.

10. Committee on Nutrition. Nutritional aspects of vegetarianism, health food, and fad diets. *Am Acad Pediat* 59, no. 3:460-64, 1977.

11. Position paper on the vegetarian approach to eating. *J Am Dietetic Assn* 77:61-69, 1980.

12. T Thom, National Heart-Lung Institute, Department of Statistics, NIH, Bethesda, MD, telephone conversation with author, April 1987.

13. Sacks FM, Donner A, Castelli WP, et al: Effect of ingestion of meat on plasma cholesterol of vegetarians. *JAMA* 246, no. 6:640-44, 1981.

14. Haines AP, Chakrabarti R, Fisher D, et al: Haemostatic variables in vegetarians and non-vegetarians. *Thrombosis Res* 19:139-48, 1980.

15. West RO, Hayes OB: A comparison between vegetarians and non-vegetarians in a Seventh-Day Adventist group. *Am J Clin Nutr* 21, no. 8:853-62, 1968.

16. Fernandes J, Dukhuis-Stoffelsma R, Groot PHE, et al: The effect of a virtually cholesterol-free, high linoleic acid vegetarian diet on serum lipoproteins of children with familial hypercholesterolemia (type II-A). *Acta Paed Scand* 70:677-82, 1981.

17. Plasma lipids and lipoproteins in vegetarians and controls. *Nutr Rev* 33, no. 9:285-86, 1975.

18. Ruys J, Hickie JB: Serum cholesterol and triglyceride levels in Australian adolescent vegetarians. *Brit Med J* 2:87, 1976.

19. Hill P, Wynder E, Garbaczewski L, et al: Plasma hormones and lipids in men at different risk for coronary heart disease. *Am J Clin Nutr* 33:1010-18, 1980.

20. Phillips RL, Lemon FR, Beeson WL, Kuzma JW: Coronary heart disease mortality among Seventh-Day Adventists with differing dietary habits: A preliminary report. *Am J Clin Nutr* 31:S191-98, 1978.

21. Sacks FM, Castelli WP, Donner A, Kass EH: Plasma lipids and lipoproteins in vegetarians and controls. *New Engl J Med* 292:1148-51, 1975.

22. Burslem J, Schonfeld G, Howald MA, et al: Plasma apoprotein and lipoprotein lipid levels in vegetarians. *Metabolism* 27, no. 6:711-19, 1978.

23. Burr ML, Sweetnam PM: Vegetarianism, dietary fiber and mortality. *Am J Clin Nutr* 36:873-77, 1982.

24. Shultz TD, Leklem JE: Dietary status of Seventh-Day Adventists and non-vegetarians. *J Am Dietetic Assn* 83, no. 1:27-33, 1983.

25. Snowdon DA, Phillips RL, Fraser GE: Meat consumption and fatal ischemic heart disease. *Prev Med* 13:490-500, 1984.

26. Moore MC, Guzman MA, Schilling PE, Strong JP: Dietary-atherosclerosis study on deceased persons. *J Am Dietetic Assn* 68:216-23, 1976.

27. Moore MC, Guzman MA, Schilling PE, Strong JP: Dietary-atherosclerosis study on deceased persons. *J Am Dietetic Assn* 79:668-72, 1981.

28. Kritchevsky, D: Vegetable protein and atherosclerosis. *J Am Oil Chem Soc* 56, no. 3:135-46, 1979.

29. Masarei JRL, Rouse IL, Lynch WJ, et al: Vegetarian diets, lipids and cardiovascular risk. *Aust N Z J Med* 14:400-404, 1984.

30. Sacks FM, Rosner B, Kass EH: Blood pressure in vegetarians. *Am J Epidemiol* 100, no. 5:390-98, 1974.

31. Abdulla M, Andersson I, Asp NG, et al: Nutrient intake and health status of vegans: Chemical analysis of diets using the duplicate portion sampling technique. *Am J Clin Nutr* 34:2464-77, 1981.

32. Abdulla M, Aly KO, Andersson I, et al: Nutrients intake and health status of lactovegetarians: Chemical analyses of diets using the duplicate portion sampling technique. *Am J Clin Nutr* 40:325-38, 1984.

33. Ophir O, Peer G, Gilad J, et al: Low blood pressure in vegetarians: The possible role of potassium. *Am J Clin Nutr* 37:755-62, 1983.

34. Margetts BM, Beilin LJ, Armstrong BK, Vandongen R: A randomized control trial of a vegetarian diet in the treatment of mild hypertension. *Clin Exper Pharm Physiol* 12:263-66, 1985.

35. Wissler R, Vesselinovitch D: Regression of atherosclerosis in experimental animals and man. *Mod Concepts Cardiovasc Dis* 46:28-29, 1977.

36. Kempner W, Peschel RL, Schlayer C: Effect of rice diet on diabetes mellitus associated with vascular disease. *Postgrad Med* 359-71, Oct 1958.

37. Pritikin N, Kaye SM, Pritikin R: Diet and exercise as a total therapeutic regimen for the rehabilitation of patients with severe peripheral vascular disease. (Paper presented at the 52nd annual session of Rehabilitation Medicine and the 37th annual assembly of the American Academy of Physical Medicine and Rehabilitation, Atlanta, GA, 19 Nov 1975) 9.

38. Wynder EL, Gori GB: Contribution of the environment to cancer incidence: An epidemiologic exercise. *J Natl Canc Inst* 58:825-32, 1977.

39. Phillips RL: Role of life style and dietary habits in risk of cancer among Seventh-Day Adventists. *Canc Res* 35:3513-22, 1975.

40. Werther JL: Does life style cause cancer? II. *N Y State J Med* 1401-08, August 1980.

41. Gori GB: Dietary and nutritional implications in the multifactorial etiology of certain prevalent human cancers. *Cancer* 43:2151-61, 1979.

42. Drasar BS, Irving D: Environmental factors in cancer of the colon and breast. *Brit J Canc* 27:167, 1973.

43. Howell MA: Diet as an etiological factor in the development of cancers of the colon and rectum. *J Chron Dis* 28:67, 1975

44. Haenszel W, Bly JW, Segi M, et al: Large bowel cancer in Hawaiian Japanese. *J Natl Canc Inst* 51:1765, 1973.

45. Manousos O, Day NE, Trichopoulous D, et al: Diet and colorectal cancer: A case-control study in Greece. *Internl J Canc* 32:1-5, 1983.

46. Berg JW, Howell MA: The geographic pathology of bowel cancer. *Cancer* 34:807-14, 1974.

47. Bosland MC: Diet and cancer of the prostate: Epidemiologic and experimental evidence, in Reddy BS, Cohen LA (eds): *Diet, Nutrition, and Cancer: A Critical Evaluation,* vol. 1. Boca Raton, FL, CRC Press, 1986, p. 142.

48. Snowdon DA, Phillips RL: Does a vegetarian diet reduce the

occurrence of diabetes? *Am J Publ Health* 75, no. 5:507-12, 1985.

49. Story L, Anderson JW, Chen WJ, et al: Adherence to high-carbohydrage, high-fiber diets: Long-term studies of non-obese diabetic men. *J Am Dietetic Assn* 85, no. 9:1105-10, 1985.

50. Jenkins DJA, Wolever TMS, Taylor RH, et al: Exceptionally low blood glucose response to dried beans: Comparison with other carbohydrate foods. *Brit Med J* 578-80, 30 Aug 1980.

51. Jenkins DJA, Wolever TMS, Jenkins AL, et al: The glycaemic index of foods tested in diabetic patients: A new basis for carbohydrate exchange favoring the use of legumes. *Diabetol* 24:257-64, 1983.

52. Jenkins DJA, Jenkins AL, Wolever TMS, et al: The glycaemic response to carbohydrate foods. *Lancet* 18 Aug 1984, 388-91.

53. Ellis F, Pathol FRC, Holesh S, Ellis J: Incidence of osteoporosis in vegetarians and omnivores. *Am J Clin Nutr* 25:555-58, June 1972.

54. Marsh AG, Sanchez TV, Mickelsen O, et al: Cortical bone density of adult lacto-ovo-vegetarian and omnivorous women. *J Am Dietetic Assn* 76:148-51, 1980.

55. Manousos O, Day NE, Tzonou A, et al: Diet and other factors in the aetiology of diverticulosis: An epidemiological study in Greece. *Gut* 26:544-49, 1985.

56. Hepner GW: Altered bile acid metabolism in vegetarians. *Digest Dis Sciences* 20:935-40, 1975.

57. Pixley F, Wilson D, McPherson K, Mann J: Effect of vegetarianism on development of gall stones in women. *Brit Med J* 291:11, 1985.

58. Sanders TAB, Ellis FR, Path FRC, Dickerson JWT: Studies of vegans: The fatty acid composition of plasma choline phosphoglycerides, erythrocytes, adipose tissue, and breast milk, and some indicators of susceptibility to ischemic heart disease in vegans and omnivore controls. *Am J Clin Nutr* 31:805-13, 1973.

59. Brown PT, Bergon JG: The dietary status of "new" vegetarians. *J Am Dietetic Assn* 67:455-59, 1975.

60. Tartter PI, Papatestas AE, Ioannovich J, et al: Cholesterol and obesity as prognostic factors in breast cancer. *Cancer* 47:2222-27, 1981.

61. Zumoff B, Dasgupta I: Relationship between body weight and the incidence of positive axillary nodes at mastectomy for breast cancer. *J Surg Oncol* 22:217, 1983.

62. National Academy of Sciences, National Research Council, Food and Nutrition Board: *Recommended Dietary Allowances,* 9th ed. Washington DC, 1980.

63. U.S. Department of Agriculture: *Nutrient Intakes: Individuals in 48 States, Year 1977-78.* Nationwide Food Consumption Survey, 1977-78, Report no. 1-2, 1984, pp. 24-25, 37-39.

64. Schroeder HA: *The Trace Elements and Man.* Old Greenwich, CT, Devin-Adair, 1973, pp. 66-84.

65. Davidson S, Passmore R, Brock JF, Truswell AS: *Human*

Nutrition and Dietetics, 7th ed. New York, Churchill Livingstone, 1979, p. 225.

66. Begley S: Silent Spring Revisited? *Newsweek,* 14 Jul 1986, 72-73.

67. Coffin DE, McKinley WP: Sources of pesticide residues, in Graham HD (ed): *The Safety of Foods,* 2nd ed. Westport, CT, AVI Publishing Co., 1980, pp. 506-11.

68. Corbett TH: *Cancer and Chemicals.* Chicago, Nelson-Hall, 1977, p. 120.

69. Ibid., p. 145.

70. Palmer S, Bakshi K: Diet, nutrition and cancer: Directions for research, in Reddy BS, Cohen LA (eds): *Diet, Nutrition, and Cancer: A Critical Evaluation,* vol. 2. Boca Raton, FL, CRC Press, 1986, p. 164.

71. Schroeder HA: *The Poisons Around Us.* Bloomington, Indiana University Press, 1974, pp. 37-56.

72. Gale NL, Wixson BG: Continued evaluation of lead in fish and mussels in the Big River of Southeastern Missouri, in Hemphill DD (ed): *Trace Substances in Environmental Health XIX.* Columbia, MO, University of Missouri, 1985, pp. 277-387.

73. Ershoff BG, Thurston EW: Effects of diet on amaranth (FD&C Red No. 2) toxicity in the rat. *J Nutr* 104:937-42, 1974.

74. Noren K: Levels of organochlorine contaminants in human milk in relation to the dietary habits of the mothers. *Acta Paed Scand* 72:811-16, 1983.

75. *Encyclopedia Americana,* s.v. "vegetarianism." New York, Grolier, 1983.

76. Fisher I: The influence of flesh eating on endurance. *Yale Med J* 13, no. 5:205-21, 1907.

77. Sussman V: *The Vegetarian Alternative.* Emmaus, PA, Rodale, 1978, p. 126.

78. *Encyclopaedia Britannica,* 1968 ed, s.v. "Olympic games."

79. Sussman, *Vegetarian Alternative,* p. 127.

80. Newnham B: Wow, like let's really try to win. *Sports Illustrated,* 12 Oct 1970, 50-51.

Commentarial Notes

nt. 1 The level of high-density lipoproteins (HDL) is also usually lowered to some extent by a vegetarian diet, but the level of low-density lipoproteins (LDL) is lowered more markedly. Since risk is generally considered to be related to the HDL/LDL ratio, the overall effect of the vegetarian diet is positive.

nt. 2 This issue is complicated by the fact that norms are often based on the intake or the body levels of the general population, so widespread deficiencies can come to be defined as normal.[62] It's possible that optimal intakes would be higher than official recommendations. Nevertheless, using Recommended Dietary Allowances (RDA) as a standard, a large percentage of the population is deficient in a number of important nutrients. (See table below.) On 10 out of 11 of these counts, the vegetarian diet was found to provide improvement.[63] Though they were not studied here, evidence suggests that a number of other nutrients, such as vitamin D (see Phase 2), pantothenic acid, zinc,[62] and chromium,[64] also may be commonly deficient.

Percentage of Individuals with Nutrient Intakes at Specified Levels of 1980 RDA

	Percentage of Individuals			
Nutrient	*Below 50% of RDA*	*50-69% of RDA*	*70-99% of RDA*	*100% and over of RDA*
Calcium	21.2	20.3	26.4	32.1
Iron	13.8	18.9	24.7	42.7
Magnesium	13.3	24.9	36.2	25.6
Phosphorus	2.1	5.4	19.3	73.3
Vitamin A	17.1	13.9	19.1	49.9
Thiamin	5.2	11.5	28.3	55.0
Riboflavin	3.7	8.4	21.9	66.0
Preformed niacin	2.5	6.6	23.8	67.1
Vitamin B_6	23.4	27.1	29.7	19.8
Vitamin B_{12}	6.2	8.8	18.5	66.5
Vitamin C	15.3	10.9	14.6	59.2

Source: Nutrient Intakes,[63] *p. 24.*

nt. 3 This study[74] was done on three groups of women: those who ate a meat-based diet, those who ate meat and fish from the Baltic, and lactovegetarians. Though the levels of the different residues varied, generally fish-eaters had the highest levels, meat-eaters intermediate levels, and lactovegetarians the least. Figures for this graph were computed by taking averages of all nonvegetarians for DDT residues plus PCBs and comparing these with similar averages for vegetarians. Other pesticide residues showed similar trends, but the differences were less pronounced.

Phase 1: Red Meat

Citational Notes

1. Schell O: *Modern Meat.* New York, Vintage, 1984, p. 197.

2. Ibid., p. 154.

3. Ibid., p. 157.

4. Tufts University: Toxic chemicals in our meat supply? *Diet and Nutrition Letter* 1, no. 3:1, 1983.

5. Schell, *Modern Meat*, p. 309.

6. Tufts University: Toxic chemicals, 1.

7. Schell, *Modern Meat*, p. 323.

8. Murrell KD, Fayer R, Dubey JP: Parasitic organisms, in Pearson AM, Dutson TR (eds): *Advances in Meat Research.* Westport, CT, AVI Publishing, 1986, pp. 311-20.

9. McClure JA: *Meat Eaters Are Threatened.* New York, Pyramid, 1973, pp. xiii, 21-22, 50.

10. Ibid., pp. 42-43.

11. Hayes W, in Ayres J, et al (eds): *Chemical and Biological Hazards in Food.* New York, Hafner, 1969, p. 144.

12. National Academy of Sciences, National Research Council, Food and Nutrition Board: *Meat and Poultry Inspection: The Scientific Basis of the Nation's Program.* Washington, DC, 1985, p. 25.

13. Schell, *Modern Meat,* p. 118.

14. Ibid., p. 23.

15. Levy SB: Man, animals and antibiotic resistance. *Pediat Infec Dis* 4, no. 1:3-5, 1985.

16. Lyons RW, Samples CL, DeSilva HN, et al: An epidemic of resistant *Salmonella* in a nursery: Animal to human spread. *JAMA* 243:546-47, 1980.

17. Siegel D, Huber WG, Drysdale S: Human therapeutic and agricultural uses of antibacterial drugs and resistance of the enteric flora of humans. *Antimicrobial Agents and Chemotherapy* 8:538-88, 1976.

18. Levy SB, Fitzgerald GB, Macone AB: Changes in the intestinal flora of farm personnel after the introduction of a tetracycline-supplemented feed on a farm. *New Engl J Med* 295:583-88, 1976.

19. Levy SB: Microbial resistance to antibiotics. *Lancet* 10 Jul 1982, 83-88.

20. National Academy of Sciences, *Meat and Poultry Inspection,* p. 27.

21. NBC Nightly News, 6 Jun 1986. New York, NBC News Archives.

22. Ben Werner, M.D., California State Department of Health Services, telephone conversation with author, 14 Jul 1986.

23. Holmberg SD, Osterholm MT, Senger CA, Cohen ML: Drug-resistant salmonella from animals fed antimicrobials. *New Engl J Med* 311:617-22, 1984.

24. Silliker JH, Gabis DA: Salmonella, in Pearson and Dutson, *Advances in Meat Research*, p. 219.

25. Watt BK, Merrill AL: *Handbook of the Nutritional Contents of Foods.* New York, Dover, 1975.

26. U.S. Department of Agriculture: *Nutrient Intakes: Individuals in 48 States, Year 1977-78.* Nationwide Food Consumption Survey, 1977-78, Report no. 1-2, 1984, p. 38.

27. Hardinge MG, Stare FJ: Nutritional studies of vegetarians, II: Dietary and serum levels of cholesterol. *J Clin Nutr* 2, no. 2:83-88, 1954.

28. Brody JE: Expert panel on cancer issues guidelines on diet. *New York Times,* 17 Jun 1982, sec. B, p. 13.

29. Rose DP, Boyar AP: Dietary fat and cancer risk: The rationale for intervention, in Reddy BS, Cohen LA (eds): *Diet, Nutrition, and Cancer: A Critical Evaluation,* vol. 1. Boca Raton, FL, CRC Press, 1986, pp. 151-56.

30. Doll R, Peto R: The causes of cancer: Quantitative estimates of avoidable risks of cancer in the United States today. *J Natl Canc Inst* 66:1192, 1981.

31. Dales LG, Friedman GD, Wry HK, et al: Case-control study of relationships of diet and other traits to colorectal cancer in American Blacks. *Am J Epidemiol* 109:132, 1979.

32. Burkitt DP, Walker AR, Painter NS: Effect of dietary fiber of stools and transit times and its role in the causation of disease. *Lancet* 2:1408, 1972.

33. Wynder EL: The epidemiology of large bowel cancer. *Canc Res* 35:3388, 1975.

34. Carroll KK: The role of dietary fat in carcinogenesis, in Perkins EG, Visek WJ (eds): *Dietary Fats and Health.* Champaign, IL, American Oil Chemists' Society, 1983, p. 710.

35. Reddy BS: Diet and colon cancer: Evidence from human and animal model studies, in Reddy and Cohen, *Diet, Nutrition, and Cancer,* vol. 1, p. 48.

36. Haenszel W, Berg JW, Segi M, et al: Large bowel cancer in Hawaiian Japanese. *J Natl Canc Inst* 51:1765-79, 1973.

37. Leveille GA: Issues in human nutrition and their probable impact on foods of animal origin. *J Animal Science* 41:723-31, 1975.

38. Carroll KK, Khor HT: Effects of level and type of dietary fat on incidence of mammary tumors induced in female Sprague-Dawley rats by 7,12-dimethylbenz (alpha) anthracene. *Lipids* 6:415, 1971.

39. Miller AB, Kelly A, Choi NW, et al: A study of diet and breast cancer. *Am J Epidemiol* 107, no. 6:499-509, 1978.

40. Hirayama T: Epidemiology of breast cancer with special reference to the role of diet. *Prev Med* 7:173-95, 1978.

41. Armstrong B, Doll R: Environmental factors and cancer incidence and mortality in different countries, with special reference to dietary practices. *Internatl J Canc* 15:617-31, 1975.

42. Carroll KK, Gammal EB, Plunkett ER: Dietary fat and mammary cancer. *Canadian Med Assn J* 98, no. 12:590-94, 1968.

43. Drasar BS, Irving D: Environmental factors and cancer of the colon and breast. *Brit J Canc* 27:167, 1973.

44. Armstrong and Doll, Environmental factors, 617.

45. Carroll KK: Experimental evidence of dietary factors and hormone-dependent cancers. *Canc Res* 35:3374, 1975.

46. Visek WJ, Clinton SK: Dietary fat and breast cancer, in Perkins and Visek, *Dietary Fats and Health*, p. 735.

47. Ibid., p. 732.

48. Burch GE: Pork and hypertension. *Am Heart J* 86, no. 5:713-14, 1973.

49. Sacks FM, Donner A, Costelli WP, et al: Effect of ingestion of meat on plasma cholesterol of vegetarians. *JAMA* 246, no. 6:640-44, 1981.

50. Newman WP, Freedman DS, Voors AW, et al: Relation of serum lipoprotein levels and systolic blood pressure to early atherosclerosis. *New Engl J Med* 314:138-44, 1986.

51. Stamler J: Lifestyles, major risk factors, proof and public policy. *Circulation* 58:1, 1976.

52. Ballentine RM: The role of nutrition in atherogenesis and acute myocardial infarction, in Califf RM, Wagner GS (eds): *Acute Coronary Care: Principles and Practice*. Boston, Martinus Nijhoff, 1985, pp. 121-33.

53. Williams RR, Hasstedt SJ, Wilson DE, et al: Evidence that men with familial hypercholesterolemia can avoid early coronary death. *JAMA* 255, no. 2:219-24, 1986.

54. Wissler K, Visselinovitch D: Regression of atherosclerosis in experimental animals and man. *Mod Concepts Cardiovasc Dis* 46:28-29, 1977.

55. Kempner W, Peschel RL, Schlayer C: Effect of rice diet on diabetes mellitus associated with vascular disease. *Postgrad Med* 359-71, Oct 1958.

56. Carroll KK: Dietary protein in relation to plasma cholesterol levels and atherosclerosis. *Nutr Rev* 36:1-5, 1978.

57. Carroll KK, Huff MW: Dietary protein and cardiovascular diseases: Effects of dietary protein on plasma cholesterol levels and cholesterol metabolism, in Santos W, Lopes N, Barbossa JJ, et al (eds): *Nutrition and Food Science*, vol. 3. New York, Plenum, 1980, pp. 378-85.

58. Moore MC, Guzman MA, Schilling PE, Strong JP: Dietary-atherosclerosis study on deceased persons. *J Am Dietetic Assn* 68:216-23, 1976.

59. Moore MC, Guzman MA, Schilling PE, Strong JP: Dietary-atherosclerosis study on deceased persons. *J Am Dietetic Assn* 79:668-72, 1981.

60. Brenner BM, Meyer TW: Dietary protein intake and the

progressive nature of kidney disease. *New Engl J Med* 307:652-54, 1982.

61. National Academy of Sciences, National Research Council, Food and Nutrition Board: *Recommended Dietary Allowances,* 9th ed. Washington, DC, 1980, pp. 16-30.

62. Michaelis OE, Ellwood KC, Judge JM, et al: Effect of dietary sucrose on the SHR/N-corpulent rat: A new model for insulin-independent diabetes. *Am J Clin Nutr* 39:612-18, 1984.

63. Jenkins DJA, Jenkins AL: Dietary fiber and the glycemic response. *Proc Soc Exper Biol Med* 180:422-31, 1985.

64. Vachon C, Jones JD, Wood PJ, et al: Improvement of glucose metabolism by soluble fibers in the rat. *Am J Clin Nutr* 43, no. 6: abst 125, 1986.

65. McArdle WD, Magel JR: Weight management: Diet and exercise, in Bland J (ed): *Medical Applications of Clinical Nutrition.* New Canaan, CT, Keats, 1983, pp. 109-110.

66. Davidson S, Passmore R, Brock JF, Truswell AS: *Human Nutrition and Dietetics,* 7th ed. New York, Churchill Livingstone, 1979, p. 251.

67. Porikos K, Hagamen S: Is fiber satiating? Effects of a high fiber preload on subsequent food intake of normal-weight and obese young men. *Appetite* 7:153-62, 1986.

68. Grimes DS, Gordon C: Satiety value of wholemeal and white bread. *Lancet* 2:106, 1978.

69. Heaton, WW: Food intake regulation and fiber, in Spiller GA, Kay RM (eds): *Medical Aspects of Dietary Fiber,* New York, Plenum, 1980, p. 227.

70. Silman A, Marr J: A better Western diet: What can be achieved? in Trowell H, Burkitt D, Heaton K (eds): *Dietary Fiber, Fiber-Depleted Foods and Disease.* New York, Academic Press, 1985, p. 410.

71. Russ CS, Atkinson RL: Use of high fiber diet for the out-patient treatment of obesity. *Nutr Reports Internatl* 32:193-98, 1985.

72. Russ CS, Atkinson RL: No effect of dietary fiber in weight loss in obesity. *Am J Clin Nutr* 43, no. 6: abst 136, 1986.

73. McClure, *Meat Eaters Are Threatened,* pp. 21, 76-77.

74. Consensus Conference. Lowering blood cholesterol to prevent heart disease. *JAMA* 253, no. 14:2080-86, 1985.

75. Brody, Expert panel on cancer.

76. Rose and Boyar, Dietary fat and cancer risk, p. 160.

77. Armstrong and Doll, Environmental factors and cancer incidence.

78. Drasar BS, Irving D: Environmental factors in cancer of the colon and breast. *Brit J Canc* 27:167, 1973.

79. Padover SL: *The Writings of Thomas Jefferson.* New York, Heritage Press, 1967.

80. Truesdell DD, Whitney EN, Acosta PB: Nutrients in vegetarian foods. *J Am Dietetic Assn* 84:28-36, 1984.

81. U.S. Department of Agriculture: *Nutritive Value of American Foods.* Agricultural handbook no. 456, 1975.

82. Davidson et al, *Human Nutrition and Dietetics,* pp. 100-2.

83. Monsen ER, Hallberg L, Layrisse M, et al: Estimation of available dietary iron. *Am J Clin Nutr* 31:134-41, 1978.

84. International Nutritional Anemia Consultative Group [cited hereafter as INACG]: *The Effects of Cereals and Legumes on Iron Availability.* Washington, DC, Nutrition Foundation, 1982, pp. 16-19.

85. Heinrich HC, Gabbe EE, Ičagić F: Nutritional iron deficiency anemia in lacto-ovo-vegetarians. *Klinische Wochenschrift* 57:187-93, 1979.

86. Dwyer JT, Dietz WH, Andrews EM, Suskind RM: Nutritional status of vegetarian children. *Am J Clin Nutr* 35:204-16, 1982.

87. Hardinge, MG, Stare, FJ: Nutritional studies of vegetarians, I: Nutritional, physical, and laboratory studies. *J Clin Nutr* 2, no. 2:73-82, 1954.

88. Shinwell ED, Gorodischer R: Totally vegetarian diets and infant nutrition. *Pediatrics* 70, no. 4:582-86, 1982.

89. Hallberg L: Iron, in *Present Knowledge in Nutrition,* 5th ed. Washington, DC, Nutrition Foundation, 1984, p. 468.

90. INACG, *Effects of Cereals and Legumes,* p. 8.

91. Cook JD, Noble NL, Morck TA, et al: Effect of fiber on nonheme iron absorption. *Gastroenterol* 85:1354-58, 1983.

92. INACG, *Effects of Cereals and Legumes,* p. 19.

93. Vyhmeister IB, Register UD, Sonnenberg LM: Safe vegetarian diets for children. *Pediat Clinics North Am* 24, no. 11:203-10, 1977.

94. James WPT: Dietary fiber and mineral absorption, in Spiller GA, McPherson R (eds): *Medical Aspects of Dietary Fiber.* New York, Plenum, 1980, p. 255.

95. Walker ARP, Walker BF: Effect of wholemeal and white bread on iron absorption. *Brit Med J* 2:771-72, 1977.

96. Bitar K, Reinhold JG: Phytase and alkaline phosphatase activities in intestinal mucosae of rat, chicken, calf, and man. *Biochimica et Biophysica Acta* 268:442-52, 1972.

97. Simpson KM, Morris ER, Cook JD: The inhibitory effect of bran on iron absorption in man. *Am J Clin Nutr* 34:1469-78, 1981.

98. Hallberg L, Rossander L: Improvement of iron nutrition in developing countries: Comparison of adding meat, soy protein, ascorbic acid, citrid acid, and ferrous sulphate on iron absorption from a simple Latin American-type of meal. *Am J Clin Nutr* 39:577-83, 1984.

99. INACG, *Effects of Cereals and Legumes,* pp. 26, 41.

100. Majumder SK: Vegetarianism: Fad, faith, or fact? *Am Scientist* 60: March/April 1972, 175-79.

101. INACG, *Effects of Cereals and Grains,* p. 9.

102. Martinez FE, Vannucchi H: Bioavailability of iron added to the diet by cooking foods in an iron pot. *Nutr Res* 6, no. 4:421-28, 1986.

103. Moore CV: Iron nutrition and requirements. *Series Haematol* 6:1-14, 1965.

104. White P: *Let's Talk About Food.* Acton, MA, Publishing Sciences Group, 1974, p. 211.

105. Sanders TA, Purves R: An anthropometric and dietary assessment of the nutritional status of vegan preschool children. *J Human Nutr* 35:349-57, 1981.

106. Abdulla M, Andersson I, Asp NG, et al: Nutrient intake and health status of vegans: Chemical analysis of diets using the duplicate portion sampling technique. *Am J Clin Nutr* 34:2464-77, 1981.

107. Bull NL, Barger SA: Food and nutrient intakes of vegetarians in Britain. *Human Nutr: Appl Nutr* 38A:288-93, 1984.

108. Harland BF, Petersen M: Nutritional status of lacto-ovo-vegetarian Trappist monks. *J Am Dietetic Assn* 72:259-64, 1978.

109. Abdulla M, Aly KO, Andersson I, et al: Nutrient intake and health status of lactovegetarians: Chemical analyses of diets using the duplicate portion sampling technique. *Am J Clin Nutr* 40:325-38, 1984.

110. Register UD, Sonnenberg LM: The vegetarian diet. *J Am Dietetic Assn* 62:253-61, 1973.

111. Anderson BM, Gibson RS, Sabry JH: The iron and zinc status of long-term vegetarian women. *Am J Clin Nutr* 34:1042-48, 1981.

112. Murray MJ, Murray AB, Murray MB, Murray CJ: The adverse effect of iron repletion on the course of certain infections. *Brit Med J* 2:1113-15, 1978.

113. Sullivan JL: Iron and the sex difference in heart disease risk. *Lancet* 1:1293-94, 1981.

114. Pollitt E, Saco-Pollitt C, Leibel RL, Viteri FE: Iron deficiency and behavioral development in infants and preschool children. *Am J Clin Nutr* 43:555-65, 1986.

115. Alberts J, Dawson EB, McGanity WJ: Affect of elevated prenatal iron supplementation on serum copper, zinc, and selenium levels. *Am J Clin Nutr* 43, no. 4: abst 673, 1986.

116. Harris M: The 100,000 year hunt. *The Sciences* 22-32, Jan/Feb 1986.

117. Sussman V: *The Vegetarian Alternative.* Emmaus, PA, Rodale, 1978, pp. 136-38.

118. Ballentine, R: *Diet and Nutrition.* Honesdale, PA, Himalayan Institute, 1982, pp. 121-23.

119. Jensen L: *Man's Foods.* Champaign, IL, Garrard Press, 1953, p. 39.

Commentarial Notes

nt. 1 The frequency with which livestock is infected has also been underestimated. Current figures, based on multiple surveys around the world, reflect an average infection rate of 20% to 30% of cows, pigs, and sheep.[8]

nt. 2 In one instance a resistant salmonella strain traveled from sick calves to the members of a farm family, and from them into a hospital nursery.[16] It has only recently been recognized that resistant organisms frequently spread from farm animals to those who work on the farm, probably by means of inhaled dust.[17,18]

nt. 3 Mung beans or spinach, as consumed, may have more fat than indicated here since the fat content of the prepared food changes as a result of the fats or oils used in cooking. Thus mung beans made according to the recipe on p. 140 will have 28% of the calories as fat. Although the lavish use of cooking fat could elevate the percentage of fat calories of vegetarian foods to a level equal to that of meats, it does not generally reach levels quite that high in practice. By decreasing the amount of cooking fat, levels can be dropped below 10%, whereas with meat-based diets it is difficult or impossible to keep the fat content of the food this low, since the fat is an integral part of the meat.

nt. 4 One who is familiar with the literature published in this area may have the impression that the use of high-fiber diets for weight loss is not well supported by the research data. In fact there is ample evidence that the principle is sound,[67-70] but several attempts to translate it into a treatment program for the obese have failed. In one study it was found that overweight subjects consumed only a little more than half the fiber recommended and thus failed to lose weight, despite their having received instruction on the rationale. The researchers concluded that the prescription of fiber-rich foods for weight loss was unlikely to succeed "due to difficulties in compliance."[71] In another trial, giving the fiber separately, as a supplement, did not help with weight loss, either.[72] Nevertheless, it is the present author's clinical impression that the principle is sound, and that properly designed high-fiber vegetarian diets do promote weight loss. If the diet is well balanced, satiety results not only from the fiber, but from having fulfilled nutritional needs. Compliance is no problem if the food is skillfully prepared according to time-honored traditions of vegetarian cooking.

nt. 5 The iron content of a half-cup serving of lentils, for example, is a difficult figure to provide with precision, for values will vary markedly according to the amount of water present in the final preparation. One half cup of a thick, nearly dry lentil dish will have much more iron (and protein and carbohydrate) than one which is soupy. Figures here are for beans cooked with an average amount of water. (Lentils, ½ cup, 100 g, 72% water; green leafy vegetables, 84% to 90% water.)

nt. 6 Although some studies suggest phytates interfere significantly with iron absorption, others disagree.[91-95] Observations of populations whose diets are high in phytic acid do not confirm the results of experiments wherein phytates have blocked iron absorption.[95]

nt. 7 The additional parameters measured were serum iron, total iron binding capacity, and calculated transferrin saturation.

nt. 8 Iron absorption also varies according to one's iron stores. Those who have a generous load of iron already on board tend to absorb less than those who are depleted. The heme-iron from meat foods is absorbed more readily, but may be less subject to regulation by how much is already present in the body. The meat-free diet, then, might allow more latitude, more ability to limit iron uptake when appropriate.[83] If this turns out to be true, it would be an asset, since there is some evidence that high iron stores may increase one's liability to infection,[112] as well as increase one's susceptibility to heart disease.[113] This is an intriguing possibility and may be an indication that our ideas of optimal iron stores should be reevaluated. Though this area deserves further study, the available data do not justify the conclusion that iron depletion is a trivial matter.

nt. 9 The Japanese experience is a case in point: between 1961 and 1971 Japanese consumption of animal protein rose 37%. Worldwide, the consumption of grain by livestock is rising twice as fast as the consumption of grain by people.[116]

nt. 10 Such look-alikes appeal especially to those whose tastes are geared to conventional meat meals. Both the author and his wife, who grew up eating meat, enjoy these bean versions of old favorites, whereas our children, who are vegetarian from birth, often find them odd and unappealing. Those for whom the re-creation of familiar tastes is not an issue seem to prefer dishes that capitalize more fully on the flavors and textures of beans, grains, and vegetables rather than trying to disguise them so as to imitate meat. Nevertheless, innovations such as bean roasts and bean burgers are helpful and fun in the transitional diet.

Phase II: Poultry

Citational Notes

1. Brewster L, Jacobson M: *The Changing American Diet.* Washington, DC, Center for Science in the Public Interest, 1983, pp. 43, 80.

2. Levy SB: Man, animals and antibiotic resistance. *Pediatric Infect Dis* 4, no. 1:3-5, 1985.

3. Pearson AM, Dutson TR: *Advances in Meat Research,* vol 2. Westport, CT, AVI Publishing, 1986, p. 222.

4. Morris GK, Wells JG: Salmonella contamination in a poultry-processing plant. *Applied Microbiol* 19:795, 1970.

5. Gibbs PA, Patterson JT, Thompson JK: The distribution of *Staphylococcus aureus* in a poultry processing plant. *J Applied Bacteriol* 44:401, 1978.

6. Notermans S, Dufrenne J, Van Leeuwen WJ: Contamination of broiler chickens by *Staphyloccus aureus* during processing; incidence and origin. *J Applied Bacteriol* 52:275, 1982.

7. Thomas CJ, McMeekin TA: Contamination of broiler carcass skin during commercial processing procedures: An electron microscopic study. *Applied Environl Microbiol* 40:133, 1980.

8. Bryan FT: Poultry and poultry meat products, in International Commission on Microbiological Specifications for Foods: *Microbial Ecology of Foods,* vol. 2, *Food Commodities.* New York, Academic Press, 1980, p. 427.

9. Mulder RW, Veerkamp CH: Improvements in poultry slaughterhouse hygiene as a result of cleaning before cooling. *Poultry Science* 53:1690, 1974.

10. Grau FJ: Microbial ecology of meat and poultry, in Pearson and Dutson, *Advances in Meat Research,* p. 16.

11. Blume E: How clean is our food? *Nutrition Action News* 13, no. 6:4-6, 1986.

12. Ben Werner, M.D., California State Department of Health Services, telephone conversation with author, 12 Jun 1986.

13. Bryan FT: Miscellaneous pathogenic bacteria, in Pearson and Dutson, *Advances in Meat Research,* pp. 250-51.

14. Ibid., p. 251.

15. Smeltzer TI: Isolation of *Campylobacter jejuni* from poultry carcasses. *Australian Vet J* 57:511, 1981.

16. Robinson DA: Infective dose of *Campylobacter jejuni* in milk. *Brit Med J* 1:1584, 1981.

17. Silliker JH: Status of Salmonella—ten years later. *J Food Protection* 43:307, 1980.

18. McClure JA: *Meat Eaters Are Threatened.* New York, Pyramid, 1973, pp. 23-24, 34-36, 55.

19. Skirrow MB, Fidoe RG, Jones DM: An outbreak of presumptive food-borne *Campylobacter* entities. *J Infect Dis* 3:234, 1981.

20. Svedhem A, Kaijser B, Sjogren E: The occurrence of *Campylobacter jejuni* in fresh food and survival under different conditions. *J Hygiene* 87:421, 1981.

21. Banwart GJ: *Basic Food Microbiology.* Westport, CT, AVI Publishing, 1983, p. 289.

22. Silliker JH, Gabis DA: Salmonella, in Pearson and Dutson, *Advances in Meat Research,* p. 212.

23. Livingston-Wheeler V, Addeo EG: *The Conquest of Cancer: Vaccines and Diet.* New York, Franklin Watts, 1984.

24. Livingston-Wheeler V, Wheeler OW (eds): *The Microbiology of Cancer: Compendium.* San Diego, Livingston-Wheeler Medical Clinic, 1977.

25. Livingston-Wheeler and Addeo, *The Conquest of Cancer,* p. 113.

26. Blackburn BO, Schlater LK, Swanson MR: Antibiotic resistance of members of the genus *salmonella* isolated from chickens, turkeys, cattle and swine in the United States during October 1981 through September 1982. *Am J Vet Res* 45:1245-49, 1984.

27. Hackler LR: *In vitro* indices: Relationships to estimating protein value for the human, in Bodwell CE (ed): *Evaluation of Proteins for Humans.* Westport, CT, AVI Publishing, 1977, pp. 55-67.

28. Orr ML, Watt BK: *Amino Acid Content of Foods.* Washington, DC, U.S. Department of Agriculture, 1968.

29. Davidson S, Passmore R, Brock JF, Truswell AS: *Human Nutrition and Dietetics,* 7th ed. New York, Churchill Livingstone, 1979, p. 40.

30. Stinke FH, Hopkins DT: Complementary and supplementary. *Cereal Foods World* 28, no. 6: 338-41, 1983.

31. Dalby A, Tsai CY: Lysine and tryptophan increases during germination of cereal grains. *Cereal Chem* 53:222-26, 1976.

32. Loma Linda Medical School, Nutrition Faculty: *Life and Health.* Special Supplement. Washington, DC, Review and Herald Publishing Association, p. 30.

33. Bressani R: Protein supplementation and complementation, in Bodwell CE: *Evaluation of Proteins for Humans.* Westport, CT, AVI Publishing, 1977, pp. 217-18.

34. Grande F, Anderson JT, Keys A: Effect of carbohydrates of leguminous seeds, wheat and potatoes on serum cholesterol concentration in man. *J Nutr* 86:313-18, 1965.

35. Mathur KS, Khan MA, Sharma KD: Hypocholesterolaemic effect of Bengal gram: A long-term study in man. *Brit Med J* 30-31, 6 Jan 1968.

36. Jenkins DJA, Wong GS, Patten R, et al: Leguminous seeds in the dietary management of hyperlipidemia. *Am J Clin Nutr* 38:567-73, 1983.

37. Gori GB: Dietary and nutritional implications in the multifactorial etiology of certain prevalent human cancers. *Cancer* 43:2151-61, 1979.

38. Jenkins DJA, Wolever TMS, Jenkins AL, et al: The glycaemic index of foods tested in diabetic patients: A new basis for carbohydrate exchange favouring the use of legumes. *Diabetol* 24:257-64, 1983.

39. Moore MC, Guzman MA, Schilling PE, Strong JP: Dietary-

atherosclerosis study on deceased persons. *J Am Dietetic Assn* 79:668-72, 1981.

40. Bressani, Protein supplementation, p. 219.

41. Herbert JR: Relationship of vegetarianism to child growth in South India. *Am J Clin Nutr* 42:1246-54, 1985.

42. Dwyer JT, Dietz WH, Andrews EM, Suskind RM: Nutritional status of vegetarian children. *Am J Clin Nutr* 35:204-16, 1982.

43. Sanders TAB, Purves R: An anthropometric and dietary assessment of the nutritional status of vegan preschool children. *J Human Nutr* 35:349-57, 1981.

44. U.S. Department of Agriculture. *Nutritive Value of American Foods.* Agricultural handbook no. 456, 1975.

45. Dubin S: How to know the chemical score, III. *Res Bulletin Himalayan Inst* 4, no. 1:38-43, 1982.

46. Sanders TH: The aflatoxin crisis, in Woodroff JG (ed): *Peanuts: Production, Processing, Products,* 3rd ed. Westport, CT, AVI Publishing, 1983, p. 151.

47. Patterson DSP: Foodborne diseases: Aflatoxicosis, in Rechcigl M (ed): *CRC Handbook of Foodborne Diseases of Biological Origin.* Boca Raton, FL, CRC Press, 1983, pp. 323-51.

48. Blume E: Aflatoxin. *Nutr Action* 13:1-6, 1986.

49. Chentanez T, et al: The effects of aflatoxin B₁ given to pregnant rats on the liver, brain and the behavior of their offspring. *Nutr Reports Internatl* 34:379-86, 1986.

50. Caster WO, et al: Dietary aflatoxins, intelligence and school performance in southern Georgia. *Internatl J Vit Nutr Res* 56:291-95, 1986.

51. Marano H: The problem with protein. *New York,* 5 Mar 1979, 49-52.

52. Hegsted M: Protein needs and possible modifications of the American Diet. *J Am Dietetic Assn* 68:317-25, 1976.

53. Cheraskin E, Ringsdorf WM, Medford FH: The "ideal" daily protein intake. *J Med Assn St Alabama* 47, no. 5:44-45, 1977.

54. Register UD, Sonnenberg LM: The vegetarian diet. *J Am Dietetic Assn* 62:253-61, 1973.

55. Bender A: Chemical scores and availability of amino acids, in Porter J, Rolls B (eds): *Proteins in Human Nutrition.* New York, Academic Press, 1973, pp. 167-78.

56. National Academy of Sciences, National Research Council, Food and Nutrition Board: *Recommended Dietary Allowances,* 9th ed. Washington, DC, 1980, pp. 46-51.

57. Hegsted DM, Trulson MF, White HS, et al: Lysine and methionine, supplementation of all-vegetable diets for human adults. *J Nutr* 56:555-76, 1955.

58. Zackin J, Meredith CN, Frontera WR, Evans WJ: Protein requirements of young endurance trained men. *Am J Clin Nutr* 43, no. 6:abst 2, 1986.

59. Aykroyd WR, Doughty J: *Wheat in Human Nutrition.* Rome, Food and Agricultural Organization of the U.N., 1971, p. 19.

60. Lappé, FM: *Diet for a Small Planet.* New York, Ballantine, 1971, p. 18.

61. Brenner BM, Meyer TW, Hostetter TH: Dietary protein intake and the progressive nature of kidney disease. *New Engl J Med* 307, no. 11:652-54, 1982.

62. Robertson WG, Heyburn PJ, Peacock M, et al: The effect of high animal protein intake on the risk of calcium stone formation in the urinary tract. *Clin Science* 57:285-88, 1979.

63. Kritchevsky D, Klurfeld D: Gallstone formation in hamsters: Effect of varying animal and vegetable protein levels. *Am J Clin Nutr* 37:802-4, 1983.

64. Visek WJ: Diet and cell growth modulation by ammonia. *Am J Clin Nutr* 31:S216-20, 1978.

65. Schuette SA, Linkswiler HM: Calcium, in Nutrition Foundation: *Present Knowledge in Nutrition,* 5th ed. Washington, DC, Nutrition Foundation, 1984, pp. 400-12.

66. McKenna MJ: Hypovitaminosis D and elevated serum alkaline phosphatase in elderly Irish people. *Am J Clin Nutr* 41:101-9, 1985.

67. Nordin BEC, Baker MR, Horsman A, et al: A prospective trial of the effect of vitamin D supplementation on metacarpal bone loss in elderly women. *Am J Clin Nutr* 42:470-74, 1985.

68. Lane NE, Block DA, Jones HH, et al: Long-distance running, bone density, and osteoarthritis. *JAMA* 255, no. 9:1147-51, 1986.

69. Albanese AA: *Bone Loss: Causes, Detection and Therapy.* New York, Alan Liss, 1977, pp. 163-64.

70. Lang R: Diagnosis and treatment of osteoporosis. Lecture delivered at a conference on metabolic bone disease. Lehigh Valley Hospital, Allentown, PA, 27 Sep 1986.

71. National Academy of Sciences, *Recommended Dietary Allowances,* p. 131.

72. Morgan KJ, Stampley GL, Zabik ME, Fischer DR: Magnesium and calcium dietary intakes of the U.S. population. *J Am College Nutr* 4:195-206, 1985.

73. National Center for Health Statistics: U.S. dietary intake: National health survey, appendix 6. *Vital and Health Statistics* series 11, no. 231, March 1983, 34-36.

74. Albanese, *Bone Loss,* p. 67.

75. Davidson et al, *Human Nutrition and Dietetics,* pp. 96-97.

76. Kummerow FA: Nutrition imbalance and angiotoxins as dietary risk factors in coronary heart disease. *Am J Clin Nutr* 32:58-83, 1979.

77. Seelig MS: *Magnesium Deficiency in the Pathogenesis of Disease.* New York, Plenum, 1980, p. 3.

78. Broadfoot MA, Trenholme MA, McClinton EP, et al: Vitamin D intakes of Ontario children. *Canad Med Assn J* 94:332-40, 1966.

79. Davidson et al, *Human Nutrition and Dietetics,* p. 124.

80. Dwyer JT, Dietz WH, Hass G, Suskind R: Risk of nutritional rickets among vegetarian children. *Am J Dis Child* 133:134-40, 1979.

81. National Academy of Sciences, *Recommended Dietary Allowances*, p. 61.

82. F. A. Kummerow, Harlan E. Moore Heart Research Laboratory, University of Illinois, telephone conversation with author, 9 Mar 1987.

83. Davidson et al, *Human Nutrition and Dietetics*, pp. 94-95.

84. Bitar K, Reinhold JG: Phytose and alkaline phosphatase activities in intestinal mucosae of rats, chicken, calf and man. *Biochimica et Biophysica Acta* 268:442-52, 1972.

85. Iengar NGC, Rao YVS: Green leafy vegetables as sources of calcium. *Annals Biochem Exper Med* 12:41-52, 1952.

86. James WPT: Dietary fiber and mineral absorption, in Spiller GA, Kay RM (eds): *Medical Aspects of Dietary Fiber*. New York, Plenum, 1980, pp. 244-48.

87. Persson I, Raby K, Fønss-Bech P, Jensen E: Effect of prolonged bran administration on serum levels of cholesterol, ionized calcium and iron in the elderly. *J Am Geriatr Soc* 24:334-35, 1976.

88. James WP, Branch WJ, Southgate DA: Calcium binding by dietary fibre. *Lancet* 1:638-39, 1978.

89. Ellis FR, Holesh S, Ellis JW: Incidence of osteoporosis in vegetarians and omnivores. *Am J Clin Nutr* 25:555-58, 1972.

90. Marsh AG, Sanchez TV, Mickelsen O, et al: Cortical bone density of adult lacto-ovo-vegetarian and omnivorous women. *J Am Dietetic Assn* 76:148-51, 1980.

91. Marsh AG, Sanchez TV, Chaffee FL, et al: Bone mineral mass in adult lacto-ovo-vegetarian and omnivorous males. *Am J Clin Nutr* 37:453-56, 1983.

92. Mazess RB, Mather W: Bone mineral content of North Alaskan Eskimos. *Am J Clin Nutr* 27:916-25, 1974.

93. Schaafsma G: *The Influence of Dietary Calcium and Phosphorus on Bone Metabolism*. Ede, Netherlands, Nederlands Instituut voor Zuivelonderzoek, 1981, p. 25.

94. Williams R: *Nutrition Against Disease*. New York, Bantam, 1981, p. 301.

95. Recker, RR, Heaney RP: The effect of milk supplements on calcium metabolism, bone metabolism and calcium balance. *Am J Clin Nutr* 41:254-63, 1985.

96. Freeland-Graves JH, Bodzy PW, Eppright MA: Zinc status of vegetarians. *J Am Dietetic Assn* 77:655-61, 1980.

97. Schaafsma, *Influence of Dietary Calcium*, pp. 27-28.

98. Barzel US, Jowsey J: The effects of chronic acid and alkali administration on bone turnover. *Clin Science* 36:517, 1969.

99. Wachman A, Bernstein DS: Diet and osteoporosis. *Lancet* 1:95, 1968.

100. Schaafsma, *Influence of Dietary Calcium*, pp. 30-38.

101. Raines-Bell R, Draper HH, Tzeng DYM, et al: Physiological

responses of human adults to foods containing phosphate additives. *J Nutr* 107:42-50, 1977.

102. National Academy of Sciences, *Recommended Dietary Allowances,* pp. 126-27.

103. Peng CF, Kane JJ, Murphy ML, Straub KD: Abnormal mitochondrial oxidative phosphorylation of ischemic myocardium reversed by Ca^{2+}-chelating agents. *J Molecular Cellular Cardiol* 9:897-908, 1977.

104. Selye H: *Calciphylaxis,* Chicago, University of Chicago Press, 1962.

105. Sincock AM: Life extension in the rotifer *Mytilina brevispina* var redunca by the application of chelating agents. *J Gerontol* 30, no. 3:289, 1975.

106. Schuette and Linkswiler, Calcium, p. 403.

107. Ballentine M: *Himalayan Mountain Cookery.* Honesdale, PA, Himalayan Institute, 1976.

108. Strause S, Saltman P: The role of manganese in bone metabolism, in Kies C (ed): *Manganese Metabolism.* ACS Monograph Series, in press.

109. Raloff J: Reasons for boning up on manganese. *Science News,* 27 Sep 1986, 199.

110. Sauchelli V: *Trace Elements in Agriculture.* New York, Van Nostrand Reinhold, 1969, pp. 18-34.

111. National Academy of Sciences, *Recommended Dietary Allowances,* p. 144.

112. Thornton I, Alloway BJ: Geochemical aspects of the soil-plant-animal relationship in the development of trace element deficiency and excess. *Proc Nutr Soc* 33:257-68, 1974.

113. Koivistoinen P, Huttunen JK: Selenium in food and nutrition in Finland, an overview on research and action. *Annals Clin Res* 18, no. 1:13-17, 1986.

114. Salonen JT: Selenium and human cancer. *Annals Clin Res* 18, no 1:18-21, 1986.

115. Ip C: Selenium and experimental cancer. *Annals Clin Res* 18, no. 1:22-29, 1986.

116. Salonen JT, Huttunen JK: Selenium in cardiovascular diseases. *Annals Clin Res* 18, no 1:30-35, 1986.

117. Combs, GF, Clark LC: Can dietary selenium modify cancer risk? *Nutr Rev* 43, no. 11:325-31, 1985.

118. Saner G, Dagoglu T, Ozden T: Hair manganese concentrations in newborns and their mothers. *Am J Clin Nutr* 41:1042-44, 1985.

119. Freeland-Graves JH, Ebangit ML, Hendrikson PJ: Alterations in zinc absorption and salivary sediment zinc after a lacto-ovo-vegetarian diet. *Am J Clin Nutr* 1757-66, 1980.

120. Åkesson B, Öckerman PA: Selenium status in vegans and lactovegetarians. *Brit J Nutr* 53:199-205, 1985.

121. Gibson RS, Anderson BM, Sabry JH: The trace metal status of

a group of post-menopausal vegetarians. *J Am Dietetic Assn* 82, no. 3:246-50, 1983.

122. Hambidge KM, Hambidge C, Jacobs M, Baum JD: Low levels of zinc in hair, anorexia, poor growth, and hypogeosia in children. *Pediat Res* 6:868-74, 1972.

123. Sandstead HH: Zinc nutrition in the United States. *Am J Clin Nutr* 26:1251-60, 1973.

124. Sandstead HH, Evans GW: Zinc, in *Present Knowledge in Nutrition,* pp. 479-505.

125. Patterson KY, Holbrook JT, Bodner JE, et al: Zinc, copper and manganese intake and balance for adults consuming self-selected diets. *Am J Clin Nutr* 40S:1397-1403, 1984.

126. White HA: Zinc content and the zinc-to-calorie ratio of weighted diets. *J Am Dietetic Assn* 68:243-45, 1976.

127. Underwood EJ: *Trace Elements in Human and Animal Nutrition,* 4th ed. New York, Academic Press, 1977, pp. 219-20.

128. Sandstead HH: A brief history of the influence of trace elements on brain function. *Am J Clin Nutr* 43:293-98, 1986.

129. Hesse GW: Chronic zinc deficiency alters neuronal function of hippocampal mossy fibers. *Science* 205:1005-7, 1979.

130. Pfeiffer CC: *Mental and Elemental Nutrients.* New Caanan, CT, Keats, 1975, 238-41.

131. Haynes DC, Gershwin ME, Golub MS, et al: Studies of marginal zinc deprivation in rhesus monkeys, VI. Influence on the immunohematology of infants in the first year. *Am J Clin Nutr* 42:252-62, 1985.

132. Freeland-Graves JH, Ebangit ML, Bodzy PW: Zinc and copper content of foods used in vegetarian diets. *J Am Dietetic Assn* 77:648-54, 1980.

133. Wade S, Bleiberg F, Mosse´ A, et al: Thymulin (Zn-Facteur Thymique Serique) activity in anorexia nervosa patients. *Am J Clin Nutr* 42:275-80, 1985.

134. Anderson BM: The iron and zinc status of long-term vegetarian women. *Am J Clin Nutr* 34:1042-48, 1981.

135. Schroeder HA: *The Trace Elements and Man.* Old Greenwich, CT, Devin-Adair, 1973, pp. 64-65.

Commentarial Notes

nt. 1 These figures are for *Staph. aureus* only, a common cause of food poisoning. Since this organism is not generally present in feces, a great deal of the contamination that occurs as a result of pounding fecal material into the skin is not reflected by this figure. Feces do often carry salmonella.

nt. 2 Early research on protein rather arbitrarily took egg white as a standard. More elaborate experiments have suggested different amino acid requirements for different age groups, and committees of experts have proposed a number of different ideal profiles.[27] Probably the most widely accepted is that suggested by an FAO/WHO committee in 1973. This is the profile detailed in the table on p. 88. It is thought to be more accurate, as well as generous enough to provide for all ages. Even with a refined reference pattern, the evaluation of protein quality is not as straightforward as one might wish. Different methods give different results, so one will find frequent discrepancies in values quoted.

The two basic methods of assessment are biological and chemical. Biological tests involve feeding the protein in question to animals or humans and measuring the amount retained or used for growth. The most common biological tests are those which yield biological value (BV) and net protein utilization (NPU). Chemical tests measure the amounts of amino acids in the protein and compare them to a reference pattern or ideal. The most common system here is that which yields the "chemical score." This number is derived by calculating the amount of the essential amino acid that is most limiting and expressing it as a percentage of the amount of that amino acid present in the ideal pattern.

The chemical scores, as calculated for the proteins of common foods, will only roughly agree with the values for NPU derived from animal experiments. Chemical scores calculated using egg white as a standard are closer to values such as protein efficiency ratio (PER), which are derived from feeding experiments, than are those scores that are based on the FAO reference pattern. But that is because egg white, which is a readily available food, is used as a control or standard in feeding experiments.

In most populations of the world, mild to moderate imbalances in essential amino acids are probably of less practical importance than are excess protein intake (in the developed countries) and a deficient carbohydrate intake (in the underdeveloped countries), both of which are potent hindrances to the efficient use of protein.

nt. 3 Actually methionine is considered the only essential one, since cystine can be made from methionine. But cystine cannot be made *de novo,* and so the diet must contain either enough of it or enough methionine to make it. Since methionine is often scarce and is a frequent limiting amino acid in protein foods, the amount of cystine present becomes important. Thus it is reasonably accurate as well as much more convenient to simply consider the two together.

nt. 4 Rice may be an important exception here. Its chemical score is 80 and if a person ate enough rice to supply his entire caloric intake, he would easily get enough protein. This helps explain why rice is a frequent choice of staples for populations who must subsist for long periods on grain alone and why therapeutic rice diets have been so successful (see Phase 1, pp. 51-52) despite the fact that they require special measures to ensure an adequate intake of vitamins and minerals.

nt. 5 Germination of most common grains (except rice) increases lysine content.[31] Sprouted grains should have a better-quality protein as a result.

nt. 6 Not all grain/legume combinations are as optimally synergistic as that of wheat and lentils. As can be seen from the table on p. 89, the combination of rice and lentils, for example, is less ideal. Corn and mung beans are not a winning team either, because they are both somewhat poor in tryptophan. But if a leafy green, such as collards, is added to mung beans and corn, the result is superb.

nt. 7 Milk has a chemical score of 100. This means that all the essential amino acids are present in amounts sufficient to permit the full use of all the other, nonessential amino acids. In fact, most of the essential amino acids in milk are present in amounts exceeding what is required to use the rest of the protein. This makes milk protein an excellent supplemental protein in many cases. It is least effective with foods that are low in methionine, however, since this is the essential amino acid it has the least generous surplus of. Since wheat is well endowed with methionine, wheat and milk work nicely together to form an excellent protein—and wheat/dairy combinations are legion, even to the point of abuse.

nt. 8 With other grains, such as wheat, soy can, at least technically, play a fully complementary role, and the combination of the two is closer to that of other grains and legumes. This is because soy has a slightly less than 100% rating for methionine, while wheat has 115% of the ideal. (Soy, though, has much more lysine than wheat.) But most authorities would consider a chemical score of 98% close enough to the ideal to preclude significant benefit from protein combining. (Chicken, for example, has a score of 98 and is considered a supplement rather than a complement for grains, despite its wealth of lysine.)

On the other hand, chemical scores calculated using egg white as a standard yield quite different results, and the reader may still encounter some figures that show soy serving as a typical complementary legume with many grains.

nt. 9 If the grain were corn, the leafy green would be even more critical since it is especially rich in tryptophan, an amino acid seriously lacking in corn and bean combinations (see table on p. 89).

nt. 10 The vegetarians in this study [41] were inhabitants of Madras, a coastal city, and did report some use of fish. One might suggest that this accounts for their better growth. However, the authors of the article make comparisons between these subjects and vegetarians studied in the West, including those who eat fish, concluding that those in the West have slightly lower heights and weights than nonvegetarian children, whereas the study of the Madrasis turned up opposite findings: the vegetarians were larger.

nt. 11 Consumer advocates report that surveys show dangerous levels of aflatoxin in 2% to 3% of commercially available peanut butter in the U.S. Both peanuts and cornmeal in the southeastern U.S. are often contaminated, because of the warm, moist climate that is conducive to the growth of the mold. A higher incidence of certain cancers,[48] birth defects,[49] and mental retardation[50] have been reported in areas where the aflatoxin levels in the food are greatest.

nt. 12 Not all foods of animal origin provide good-quality protein. Gelatin, which is made from animal connective tissues, is 85% protein, but is grossly deficient in a number of the essential amino acids. It is of such a poor quality that its tryptophan level is less than 1% of the ideal— probably the lowest figure for any common foodstuff, vegetable or animal.[28]

nt. 13 When there is too much vitamin D, its efforts to increase body calcium are overdone. Not only does it increase intestinal absorption, it also holds on to calcium by preventing the kidneys from getting rid of it through the urine. Thus the overall effect of vitamin D is to *conserve* calcium, but when it is taken in excess, too much calcium is held in. In such cases, as will become apparent when parathyroid action is discussed, calcium can't get out, but it doesn't get to the bones either, because the excess vitamin D causes mobilization of calcium from bone to exceed deposition.

When vitamin D is taken in high doses over long periods, one will find bone spurs and arterial calcifications. In fact, experimental feeding of high doses of vitamin D in swine has produced advanced vascular disease that appears to be identical to human atherosclerosis. Some researchers also think that high levels of vitamin D in the blood may be one of the irritants that can damage the lining of the arteries and provoke the deposition of cholesterol in them.[76]

A rise in vitamin D intake began in the 1930s when it was added to foods in quantities that would cure, rather than merely prevent, rickets. Such fortification was made mandatory in many states, and extended from milk to margarine, breakfast cereals, and flour. The cumulative intake that became possible under these circumstances led the Committee on Nutrition of the American Academy of Pediatrics to express concern about the danger of overdose. In 1963 the committee calculated that the total intake by a child eating available foods could range from 600 IU to 4,000 IU a day.[77] A survey done the same year of 1,000 Canadian children under six years of age showed that 70% consumed more than 400 IU, and 30% consumed over 1,000 IU of vitamin D per day.[78] This must be regarded as a serious problem, since experts indicate that an

important consideration with vitamin D is the narrow gap between the
nutrient requirement and a toxic dose. As little as five times the
recommended intake (2,000 IUs) has produced symptoms of toxicity,[79]
and intakes may be exceeding that in some cases, as will be explained.

nt. 14 Though 20% to 40% of this calcium may be recovered when
cellulose is digested by the bacteria of the colon, still up to a third more
of the calcium in food is lost with cellulose feeding.[86]

nt. 15 The data in this graph are for women only. The incidence of
crippling osteoporosis is much lower in men.

nt. 16 Paradoxically, this effect may be partially countered by the
meat itself, the high phosphate content of which (through PTH—as will
be discussed) prompts the kidney to conserve calcium. Thus the
overabundance of phosphorus in meat may help prevent meat's excess of
protein from causing a loss of body calcium. But this won't benefit the
bones, since the PTH triggered by the phosphorus will demineralize
rather than strengthen bone. We might postulate, then, that calcium
balance can be maintained on a high-meat, high-phosphorus diet, but
only at the expense of bone loss.

nt. 17 Today, high doses of calcium supplements are being taken in
an effort to treat or prevent osteoporosis. When this is done in the face of
a high-phosphate diet and the resulting background of recurrent rises in
PTH, the calcium will merely be driven into the tissues, and may
overwhelm cell membrane mechanisms designed to keep it out. This
seems to be a concept that has been recognized only sporadically until
recently. Hans Selye wrote a book in 1962 that noted the accumulation of
calcium in tissues in chronic disease.[104] Currently there is a new interest in
the difference between the effects of intra- and extra-cellular calcium in
the pathogenesis of a number of diseases. The pharmaceutical industry
has recently been developing and promoting "calcium blocking agents,"
drugs that enter the cell and interfere with the activity of calcium there.
Their use is being found to provide some relief in a number of disorders
that are currently common.

nt. 18 Detailed recipes can be found in *Himalayan Mountain
Cookery.*[107]

nt. 19 In view of this, it is interesting that some cases of schizophrenia
seem to clear dramatically when given zinc.[130]

nt. 20 It is known that patients with anorexia nervosa have lowered
levels of a zinc-dependent thyroid hormone.[133] In view of the depressed
appetite observed in the Denver boys when their sense of taste waned due
to zinc deficiency, one can't help but wonder whether women, especially

those who are particularly weight-conscious, might limit themselves to low-zinc foods in part to help control their appetites. A self-induced anorexia would make it easier to resist eating, though it would be unlikely to lead to a healthy kind of thinness. In any case, whatever their reasons, the women in the zinc study were described as making "poor food choices."

nt. 21 The vegetarians in the first study[96, 131] were part of a university community and for the most part had little systematic training in vegetarian nutrition or food selection.

The situation is somewhat better in the case of Seventh-Day Adventists, for example. While these people follow a nonmeat diet for religious reasons, they are often well versed in the practical side of nutrition, having the advantage of excellent classes and publications provided by the medical professinals in their ranks. As a result, one might expect their diets to be more reasonably balanced and their foods more consistently well selected. When hair and blood levels of zinc were measured in 56 long-term Seventh-Day Adventist vegetarian women, all fell within the normal range.[134]

Phase 3: Fish

Citational Notes

1. Price W: *Nutrition and Physical Degeneration.* Santa Monica, CA, Price-Pottenger Nutrition Foundation, 1975, p. 263.
2. Brewster L, Jacobson MF: *The Changing American Diet.* Washington, DC, Center for Science in the Public Interest, 1983, pp. 24-25, 78.
3. Davidson S, Passmore R, Brock JF, Truswell AS: *Human Nutrition and Dietetics,* 7th ed. New York, Churchill Livingstone, 1979, p. 189.
4. Dyerberg J, Bang HO: Haemostatic function and platelet polyunsaturated fatty acids in Eskimos. *Lancet* 1 Sep 1979, 433-35.
5. Harai A, Terano T, Saito H, et al: Eicosapentaenoic acid and platelet function in Japanese, in Lovenberg W, Yamori Y (eds): *Nutritional Prevention of Cardiovascular Disease.* New York, Academic Press, 1984, pp. 231-39.
6. Herold PM, Kinsella JE: Fish oil consumption and decreased risk of cardiovascular disease. *Am J Clin Nutr* 43:566-98, 1986.
7. Knapp HR, Reilly IAG, Alessondrini P, Fitzgerald GA: In vivo indexes of platelet and vascular function during fish-oil administration in patients with atherosclersis. *New Engl J Med* 314, no. 15:937-42, 1986.
8. Norell S, et al: Fish consumption and mortality from coronary heart disease. *Brit Med J* 239:426, 1986.

9. von Lossonczy TO, Ruiter A, Bronsgeest-Schoute HC, et al: The effect of a fish diet on serum lipids in healthy human subjects. *Am J Clin Nutr* 31:1340-46, 1978.

10. Sanders T, Sullivan DR, Reeve J, Thompson GR: Triglyceride-lowering effect of marine polyunsaturates in patients with hypertriglyceridemia. *Arteriosclerosis* 5:459-65, 1985.

11. Singer P, Wirth M, Voigt S, et al: Blood pressure and lipid-lowering effect of mackerel and herring diet in patients with mild essential hypertension. *Atherosclerosis* 56:223-35, 1985.

12. Ballard-Barbash R, Callaway CW: Marine fish oils: Role in prevention of coronary artery disease. *Mayo Clin Proc* 62:113-18, 1987.

13. Singer P, Wirth M, Berger I, et al: Influence on serum lipids, lipoproteins and blood pressure of mackerel and herring diet in patients with Type IV and V hyperlipoproteinemia. *Atherosclerosis* 56:111-18, 1985.

14. Nettleton JA: *Seafood Nutrition.* Huntington, NY, Osprey, 1985, p. 29.

15. Puustinen T, Punnonen K, Notila P: The fatty acid composition of 12 north-European fish species. *Acta Med Scand* 218:59-62, 1985.

16. Ziemlanski S, Panczenko-Kresowska B, Okolska G, et al: Effect of dietary fats on experimental hypertension. *Ann Nutr Metab* 29:223-31, 1985.

17. Norris PG, Jones CHJ, Weston MJ: Effect of dietary supplementation with fish oil on systolic blood pressure in mild essential hypertension. *Brit Med J* 293:104-5, 1986.

18. Glueck CG, McCarren T, Hitzemann R, et al: Amelioration of severe migraine with omega-3 fatty acids: A double-blind, placebo-controlled clinical trial. *Am J Clin Nutr* 43, no. 4: abst 710, 1986.

19. Tamura Y, Hirai A, Terano T, et al: Effect of administration of highly purified eicosapentaenoic acid on platelet and erythrocyte functions in patients with thrombitic disorders, in Lovenberg and Yamori, *Nutritional Prevention of Cardiovascular Disease,* pp. 323-30.

20. Bang H, Dyerberg J: The bleeding tendency in Greenland Eskimos. *Danish Med J* 27:202-5, 1980.

21. Mead JF: Free radical mechanisms in lipid peroxidation and prostaglandins, in Armstrong D, Sohal RS, Cutler RG, Slater TF (eds): *Free Radicals in Molecular Biology, Aging, and Disease.* Aging Series, vol. 27. New York, Raven Press, 1984, p. 58.

22. Galland L: Increased requirements for essential fatty acids in atopic individuals: A review with clinical descriptions. *J Am College Nutr* 5:213-28, 1986.

23. Banwart GJ: *Basic Food Microbiology.* Westport, CT, AVI Publishing, 1983, pp. 442-43.

24. Litchfield JH: Salmonella food poisoning, in Graham HD (ed): *The Safety of Foods,* 2nd ed. Westport, CT, AVI Publishing, 1980, p. 123.

25. Banwart, *Basic Food Microbiology,* p. 297.

26. Rechcigl M: *Handbook of Nutritive Value of Processed Food*, vol. 1, *Food for Human Use*. Boca Raton, FL, CRC Press, 1984, pp. 370-72.

27. International Commission on Microbiological Specifications for Foods. *Microbial Ecology of Foods*, vol. 2, *Food Commodities*. New York, Academic Press, 1980, pp. 593-94.

28. Banwart, *Basic Food Microbiology*, p. 297.

29. Pressnell MW, Cummins JM, Miescier JJ: Influence of selected environmental factors on the elimination of bacteria by the Eastern oyster (*Crassostera virginica*), in U.S. Department of Health, Education, and Welfare, Public Health Service: *Proceedings of Gulf and South Atlantic Shellfish Sanitation Conference*. Washington, DC, 1969, pp. 47-65.

30. DiGirolamo RG: The uptake, elimination and effects of processing on the survival of polio virus in West Coast oysters. Ph.D. diss., University of Washington, 1969.

31. Janssen WA: Oysters: Retention and excretion of three types of waterborne disease bacteria. *Health Lab Science* 2, no. 1:20-24, 1974.

32. International Commission on Microbiological Specifications for Foods, *Microbial Ecology of Foods*, p. 595.

33. Cann DC: Bacteriology of shellfish with reference to international trade, in Tropical Prod. Institute, *Handling, Processing and Marketing of Tropical Fish*. London, Tropical Prod. Institute, 1977, pp. 377-94.

34. Graham, *Safety of Foods*, pp. 445-46, 449.

35. Noren K: Levels of organochlorine contaminants in human milk in relation to the dietary habits of mothers. *Acta Paed Scan* 72:811-16, 1983.

36. Weiner MA: Cholesterol in foods rich in omega-3 fatty acids. *New Engl J Med* 315:883, 1986.

37. Sunopoulos AP, Salem N: Purslane: A terrestrial source of omega-3 fatty acids. *New Engl J Med* 315:833, 1986.

38. Johnels AG, Westermark T: Mercury contamination of the environment in Sweden, in Miller MW, Berg GG (eds): *Chemical Fallout: Current Research on Persistent Pesticides*. Springfield, IL, Charles C. Thomas, 1969, pp. 221-41.

39. Borg K, Wanntorp H, Erne K, Hanko E: Mercury poisoning in Swedish wildlife. *J Appl Ecol* 3:S171-72, 1966.

40. Schroeder HA: *The Poisons Around Us*. Bloomington, IN, Indiana University Press, 1974, pp. 63-72.

41. Goldwater LJ: Mercury in the environment. *Scientific Am* 224, no. 5:15-21, 1971.

42. Underwood EJ: *Trace Elements in Human and Animal Nutrition*. New York, Academic Press, 1977, pp. 379-83.

43. Ohlson CG, Hogstedt C: Parkinson's disease and occupational exposure to organic solvents, agricultural chemicals and mercury—a case-referent study. *Scand J Work Environl Health* 7:252-56, 1981.

44. Chang LM: Mercury, in Spencer PS, Schaumburg HH (eds): *Experimental and Clinical Neurotoxicology*. New York, Williams and Wilkins, 1980, p. 512.

45. Heintze U, Edwardsson S, Derand R, Brikhed D: Methylation of mercury from dental amalgam and mercuric chloride by oral streptococci in vitro. *Scand J Dent Res* 91:150-52, 1983.

46. Shepard DAE: Methylmercury poisoning in Canada. *Canad Med Assn* 114:459-63, 1976.

47. Lommel A, Kruse H, Wasserman O: Organochlorines and mercury in blood of a fish-eating population at the River Elbe in Schleswig-Holstein, FRG. *Arch Toxicol* suppl 8:264-68, 1985.

48. Graham, *Safety of Foods,* pp. 625-51.

49. Chanarin I: The cobalamins (vitamin B_{12}), in Barker BM, Bender DA (eds): *Vitamins in Medicine,* vol. 1. London, Heinemann, 1980, pp. 172-246.

50. Jathar VS, Inamdar-Deshmukh AB, Rege DV, Satoskar RS: Vitamin B_{12} and vegetarianism in India. *Acta Haemat* 53:90-97, 1975.

51. Inamdar-Deshmukh AB, Jathar VS, Joseph DA, Satoskar RS: Erythrocyte vitamin B_{12} activity in healthy Indian lacto-vegetarians. *Brit J Haemat* 32:395-401, 1976.

52. Immerman AM: Vitamin B_{12} status on a vegetarian diet: A critical review. *World Rev Nutr Diet* 37:38-54, 1981.

53. Misra HN, Fallowfield JM: Subacute combined degeneration of the spinal cord in a vegan. *Postgrad Med J* 47:624-26, 1971.

54. Hines JD: Megaloblastic anemia in an adult vegan. *Am J Clin Nutr* 19:260-68, 1966.

55. Paige DM: *Manual of Clinical Nutrition.* Pleasantville, NJ, Nutrition Publications, 1983, p. 35.5.

56. Ellis FR, Montegriffo VME: Veganism, Clinical findings and investigations. *Am J Clin Nutr* 23:249-55, 1970.

57. Chanarin I, Malkowska V, O'Hea AM, et al: Megaloblastic anaemia in a vegetarian Hindu community. *Lancet* 23 Nov 1985, 1168-72.

58. Thomaskutty KG, Lee CM: Interaction of nutrition and infection: Effect of vitamin B_{12} deficiency on resistance to *Trypanosoma lewisi. J Natl Med Assn* 77:289-97, 1985.

59. Thrash AM, Thrash CL: *Nutrition for Vegetarians.* Seale, AL, Thrash Publications, 1982, p. 67.

60. Goodman LS, Gilman A (eds): *The Pharmacological Basis of Therapeutics.* New York, MacMillan, 1970, p. 1419.

61. U.S. Department of Agriculture: *Pantothenic Acid, Vitamin B_6 and Vitamin B_{12} in Foods.* USDA home economics research report no. 36, August 1969.

62. Shurtleff W: Sources of vegetarian vitamin B_{12}. *Vegetarian Times* May/June 1979, 36.

63. Herbert V: Vitamin B_{12}, in *Present Knowledge in Nutrition,* 5th ed. Washington, DC, Nutrition Foundation, 1984, p. 358.

64. Albert MJ, Mathan VI, Baker ST: Vitamin B_{12} synthesis by human small intestine bacteria. *Nature* 283:781-82, 1980.

65. National Academy of Sciences, National Research Council, Food and Nutrition Board: *Recommended Dietary Allowances,* 9th ed. Washington, DC, 1980, pp. 112-20.

66. Siddens RC: The experimental production of vitamin B_{12} deficiency in the baboon (*Papio cynocephalus*). A 2-year study. *Brit J Nutr* 32:219-28, 1974.

67. Lampkin BC, Saunders RF: Nutritional vitamin B_{12} deficiency in an infant. *Pediatrics* 75:1053, 1969.

68. Higginbottom MC, Sweetman L, Nyhan WL, et al: A syndrome of methylmalonic aciduria, homocystinuria, megaloblastic anemia and neurologic abnormalities in a vitamin B_{12} deficient breastfed infant of a strict vegetarian. *New Engl J Med* 299:317-23, 1978.

69. Vitamin B_{12} deficiency in the breastfed infant of a strict vegetarian. *Nutr Rev* 37, no. 5:142-44, 1979.

70. Herbert V, Jacob E: Destruction of vitamin B_{12} by ascorbic acid. *JAMA* 230:241-42, 1974.

71. Newmark HL, Scheiner J, Marcus M, Prabhudesai M: Stability of vitamin B_{12} in the presence of ascorbic acid. *Am J Clin Nutr* 29:645-49, 1976.

72. Herbert V, Jacob E, Wong K, et al: Low serum vitamin B_{12} levels in patients receiving ascorbic acid in megadoses: Studies concerning the effect of ascorbate on radioisotope vitamin B_{12} assay. *Am J Clin Nutr* 31:253-58, 1978.

73. Kondo H, Binder MK, Kolhouse JF, et al: Presence and formation of cobalamin analogues in multiple vitamin-mineral pills. *J Clin Invest* 70:889-98, 1982.

74. Herbert V, Drivas G, Foscaldi R, et al: Multivatimin/mineral food supplements containing vitamin B_{12} may also contain analogues of B_{12}. *New Engl J Med* 307:255-56, 1982.

75. Herbert V, Drivas G: Spirulina and vitamin B_{12}. *JAMA* 248, no. 23:3096-97, 1982.

76. Edozien J, Udo U, Young V, et al: Effects of high level of yeast feeding on uric acid metabolism of young men. *Nature* 228:180, 1970.

77. Ballentine, RM: *Diet and Nutrition.* Honesdale, PA, Himalayan Institute, 1978, p. 170.

78. Dalal T: *Indian Vegetarian Cookbook.* New York, Hamlyn, 1983.

79. Sahini J: *Classic Indian Vegetarian and Grain Cooking.* New York, Morrow, 1985.

80. Jaffrey M: *A Taste of India.* New York, Atheneum, 1986.

81. Ballentine M: *Himalayan Mountain Cookery: A Vegetarian Cookbook.* Honesdale, PA, Himalayan Institute, 1976.

Commentarial Notes

nt. 1 Early experiments showed a decrease in blood fats in those with seriously elevated cholesterol levels. But fish oil can also lower blood lipids in persons with average levels. For example, a total of 42 ovolactovegetarians living in a Dutch monastery and a Belgian convent were given a diet to which had been added mackerel, a rather high-fat fish. Then, for an equal length of time, they were given the same diet except with full-fat cheese replacing the fish. Comparing the fish diet with that containing cheese, there was a slight lowering of cholesterol and a more substantial lowering of triglycerides.[9] Subsequent work on fish oil has confirmed this appreciable decrease in triglycerides, while it has also demonstrated increases in high-density lipoprotein (HDL).[10-12] Some of the studies have found significant decreases in total cholesterol too, [11,12] but others have not.[10]

nt. 2 In a recent study, patients with vascular disease who were given 50 milliliters of fish oil (containing 10 grams of EPA) a day for four weeks showed an average 58% increase in bleeding time after the first week of treatment (from 3.3 minutes to 5.2 minutes).[7]

nt. 3 Though in the study of the Japanese fishing village mentioned earlier, consumption amounted to approximately ½ pound per day, the research team stated that they thought a substantially protective effect would result from half that much.[5]

nt. 4 Though red blood cells are apparently affected to some extent, the major effect seems to show up in the platelets, small cell-like bodies in the blood that are intimately involved in the formation of blood clots. Before EPA was given to patients with vascular disease, in a recent experiment, they were found to have elevated levels of a thromboxane (A_2) that promotes clotting. After EPA, this thromboxane was converted into a different one (A_3) that did not participate in the clotting process.[7] Arachidonic acid is used to make A_2, EPA to make A_3.

nt. 5 Of 85 patients, 6 were discovered to have what could be significant exposure to various forms of mercury. While this is not a statistically significant number, it is enough, when one considers the similarity of the symptoms of mercury poisoning and Parkinson's disease, to warrant further exploration. It is possible that mercury toxicity may contribute to the development of the disease in a certain subgroup of Parkinsonian patients.

nt. 6 Daily fish consumption among these people is about two thirds of a pound a day, increasing to more than twice that in the summer. Fish in northern Canada have been found to have up to 2,000 parts per billion (ppb) of mercury. Some of the Indians have shown blood levels of mercury of over 600 ppb.[46] The normal level is from 5 to 10. From experiences in mass poisonings like Minamata, it is accepted that blood levels of 1,000 ppb and over will produce a full-blown picture of toxicity with a substance like mercury, which accumulates. The 600 to 1,000 ppb range is suggestive of chronic, gradual poisoning.

nt. 7 The following criteria have been suggested:[52]

1. It must be shown that the patient has taken in less than the minimum adult requirement of about 1 microgram a day (see chart for B_{12} content of common foods). (Official RDAs are higher—this is the amount needed to prevent deficiency symptoms.)
2. The patient must have abnormally low blood levels of vitamin B_{12}.
3. It must be shown that his ability to absorb B_{12} is unimpaired. (If he can't absorb it, then his deficiency state is due to that problem, not to a lack of B_{12} in the diet.)
4. He must exhibit signs and symptoms of B_{12} deficiency: anemia or neurological degeneration.
5. These signs and symptoms must disappear when he's given oral doses of the normal daily requirements of B_{12}. If injections are necessary, then it's his absorption that's defective, not his diet.

nt. 8 More recently there is at least one study[57] that reported nutritional B_{12} deficiency in as much as 1% of East Indian immigrants to England. While this may be attributed to disruptions in the microbial ecology of the gut, as described above, it seems unlikely. The patients were mostly lactovegetarians and should have adequate intake of B_{12}. How such a large number of cases was diagnosed becomes apparent when the criteria used by the investigator are analyzed carefully. They were selected by examining the records of bone marrow aspirations done in an English hospital serving an area with a large Indian community. All those records mentioning megaloblastic hemapoiesis (red cells that are larger than average) who also had names that appeared to be East Indian were studied. This turned up 138 patients in a 14-year period. Of these, 20 had pernicious anemia, due to lack of intrinsic factor and apparently unrelated to diet, and 23 others had megaloblastic marrow due to other causes such as folic acid deficiency or anti-convulsant medication. The remaining 95 were assumed to be cases of nutritional B_{12} deficiency. Since all of these patients were sick enough to have bone marrow aspirations done, that could account for the relative deficiency of their vitamin levels. It is known that illness increases one's B_{12} needs. Other explanations besides simple dietary deficiency include, besides disruptions of gut flora by immigration, the use of antibiotics or the intake of supplements or other substances available in the U.K. that might act as B_{12} antagonists (see below). In any case it is not clear how many, if any, satisfied all the criteria mentioned above for establishing dietary B_{12} deficiency beyond all doubt.

One might conclude from such a study, however, that illness can tip the balance for the vegetarian—especially the vegan, but even the lactovegetarian. This does not necessarily mean that the vegetarian should routinely increase his intake of B_{12}, but it does suggest he should do so when ill. This is important not only to prevent the classic symptoms of pernicious anemia, but also because B_{12} deficiency has been shown to compromise the ability of white cells to destroy infecting microbes[57] and to diminish the immune response.[58]

nt. 9 Other research supports this idea. Baboons developed B_{12} deficiency when put on a refined diet low in B_{12}, but the deficiency was more severe when they were also fed antibiotics.[66]

nt. 10 Nutritional yeast is not a traditional food and might be considered experimental. It is grown under varying conditions and its quality may vary. Even the best available may create problems, especially when taken in quantity. Three tablespoons a day produced elevated levels of uric acid in healthy subjects, an effect which could precipitate attacks of gout.[76,77]

nt. 11 Because traditional Indian cooking at its best is highly improvisational, good-quality cookbooks that reflect the spirit of Indian cuisine have been slow to appear in the West. Recently, however, a number of attractive and artistic works have appeared that portray the delicacy and appeal of the food.[78-80]

Now That You're a Vegetarian

Citational Notes

1. Brisson GJ: *Lipids in Human Nutrition.* Englewood, NJ, Jack K. Burgess, 1981, p. 17.

2. Sacks FM, Costelli WP, Donner A, Kass EH: Plasma lipids and lipoproteins in vegetarians and controls. *New Engl J Med* 292, no. 22: 1148-51, 1975.

3. Liebman M, Bazzarre TL: Plasma lipids of vegetarian and non-vegetarian males: Effects of egg consumption. *Am J Clin Nutr* 38:612-19, 1983.

4. Trafford A, Carey J, Whitman D, et al: America's diet wars. *U.S. News and World Report* 20 Jan 1986, 62-66.

5. Flynn MA, Nolph GB, Flynn TC, et al: Effect of dietary egg on human serum cholesterol and triglycerides. *Am J Clin Nutr* 32:1051-57, 1979.

6. Hausman P: Unscrambling the egg controversy. *Nutr Action* 5, no. 12:3-6, 1978.

7. Brisson, *Lipids in Human Nutrition,* pp. 81-82.

8. Ballentine RM: The role of nutrition in atherogenesis and acute myocardial infarction, in Califf RM, Wagner GS (eds): *Acute Coronary Care.* Boston, Martinus Nijhoff, 1985, pp. 121-33.

9. Brisson, *Lipids in Human Nutrition,* pp. 73-94.

10. Oh SY, Miller LT: Effect of dietary egg on variability of plasma cholesterol levels and lipoprotein cholesterol. *Am J Clin Nutr* 42, no. 3: 421-31, 1985.

11. Abdulla M, Aly KO, Andersson I, et al: Nutrient intake and health status of lactovegetarians. *Am J Clin Nutr* 40:325-38, 1984.

12. Mason RL, Kunkel ME, Davis TA, et al: Nutrient intakes of vegetarian and nonvegetarian women. *Tennessee Farm Home Science,* Jan/Feb 1978, 18-20.

13. Underwood EJ: *Trace Elements in Human and Animal Nutrition.* New York, Academic Press, 1977, pp. 459-60.

14. Schroeder HA: *The Trace Elements and Man.* Old Greenwich, CT, Devin-Adair, 1973, p. 46.

15. Inglett GE, Falkehag SI (eds): *Dietary Fibers: Chemistry and Nutrition.* New York, Academic Press, 1979, p. 87.

16. Ibid., p. 268.

17. Reddy BS: Diet and colon cancer: Evidence from human and animal model studies, in Reddy BS, Cohen LA (eds): *Diet, Nutrition, and Cancer: A Critical Evaluation,* vol. 1. Boca Raton, FL, CRC Press, 1986, pp. 57-58.

18. Williams RJ: *Nutrition Against Disease.* New York, Bantam, 1981, p. 193.

19. Rao DR, Pulusani SR, Chawan CB: Natural inhibitors of carcinogenesis: Fermented milk products, in Reddy BS, Cohen LA (eds): *Diet, Nutrition, and Cancer: A Critical Evaluation,* vol. 2. Boca Raton, FL, CRC Press, 1986, p. 73.

20. Hirayama T: Epidemiology of cancer of the stomach with special reference to its recent decrease in Japan. *Canc Res* 35:3460-63, 1975.

21. Rao et al, Natural inhibitors of carcinogenesis, in Reddy and Cohen, *Diet, Nutrition, and Cancer,* vol. 1, p. 73.

22. Nair CR, Mann GV: A factor in milk which influences cholesteremia in rats. *Atherosclerosis* 26:363-67, 1977.

23. Bayless TM, Rothfeld B, Massa C, et al: Lactose and milk intolerance: Clinical implications. *New Engl J Med* 292, no. 22:1156-59, 1975.

24. Wrench GT: *The Wheel of Health.* New York, Schocken, 1972, pp. 86-87.

25. Bayless TM, Huang SS: Recurrent abdominal pain due to milk and lactose intolerance in school-aged children. *Pediatrics* 47, no. 6:1029-32, 1971.

26. Savaiano DA, AbouElAnouar A, Smith DE, Levitt MD: Lactose malabsorption from yogurt, pasteurized yogurt, sweet acidophilus milk, and cultured milk in lactase-deficient individuals. *Am J Clin Nutr* 40:1219-23, 1984.

27. Gallagher CR, Molleson AL, Caldwell JH: Lactose intolerance and fermented dairy products. *J Am Dietetic Assn* 65:418-19, 1974.

28. Locke SE, Hornig-Rohan M: *Mind and Immunity: Behavioral*

Immunology. New York, Institute for the Advancement of Health, 1983, pp. 130-42, 148-50.

29. Buisseret PD: Common manifestations of cow's milk allergy in children. *Lancet* 11 Feb 1978, 304-5.

30. Food allergy. *Lancet* 3 Feb 1979, 249-50.

31. Graham HD (ed): *The Safety of Foods.* Westport, CT, AVI Publishing, 1980, pp. 385-93.

32. Milk: Why is the quality so low? *Consumer Reports* Jan 1974, 70-76.

33. Dr. Pavia, Enteric Disease Division, Center for Disease Control, Atlanta, GA, telephone conversation with author, 28 Apr 1987.

34. G. M. Dunny, D.V.M., College of Veterinary Medicine, Cornell University, telephone conversation with author, 28 Apr 1987.

35. Agranoff BW, Goldberg D: Diet and the geographical distribution of multiple sclerosis. *Lancet* 2 Nov 1974, 1061-66.

36. Agranoff BW: Multiple sclerosis, in Perkins EG, Visek WJ (eds): *Dietary Fats and Health.* Champaign, IL, American Oil Chemists' Society, 1983, p. 947.

37. Wrench, *The Wheel of Health,* p. 100.

38. Webb BH, Johnson AH, Alford JA (eds): *Fundamentals of Dairy Chemistry.* Westport, CT, AVI Publishing, 1974, pp. 611-12.

39. Williams, *Nutrition Against Disease,* pp. 298-300.

40. Dayton S, Pearce MT, Hashimoto S, et al: A controlled clinical trial of a diet high in unsaturated fat in preventing complications of atherosclerosis. *Circulation* 40, no. 1, suppl 2:1-63, 1969.

41. Miettinen M, Turpeinen O, Karvonen MJ, et al: Effect of cholesterol-lowering diet on mortality from coronary heart disease and other causes. *Lancet* 21 Oct 1972, 835-38.

42. Morris JN, Ball KP, Antonis A, et al: Controlled trial of soybean oil in myocardial infarction. *Lancet* 28 Sep 1968, 693-700.

43. Leren P: The Oslo Diet-Heart Study. *Circulation* 42:935-42, 1970.

44. West CE, Redgrave TG: Reservations on the use of polyunsaturated fats in human nutrition. *Am Lab* Jan 1975, 23-30.

45. Pearce ML, Dayton S: Incidence of cancer in men on a diet high in polyunsaturated fat. *Lancet* 6 Mar 1971, 464-67.

46. Ederer F, Leren P, Turpeinen O, Frantz ID: Cancer among men on cholesterol-lowering diets. *Lancet* 24 Jul 1971, 203-6.

47. Mead JF: Dietary polyunsaturated fatty acids as potential toxic factors. *Chem Technol* 2, no. 2:70-71, 1972.

48. Mickel HS: Peroxidized arachidonic acid effects on human platelets and its proposed role in the induction of damage to white matter, in Kabara JJ (ed): *The Pharmacological Effects of Lipids.* Champaign, IL, American Oil Chemists Society, 1978, pp. 179-90.

49. Kaunitz H: Toxic effects of polyunsaturated vegetable oils, in Kabara, *Pharmacological Effects of Lipids,* pp. 203-10.

50. Pryor WA: Free radicals in biological systems. *Scientific Am* 223, no. 2:70-83, 1970.

51. Pryor WA, Stanley JP, Blair E, et al: Autoxidation of polyunsaturated fatty acids. *Arch Environl Health* July/August 1976, 201-10.

52. Brisson, *Lipids in Human Nutrition,* p. 8.

53. Nanji AA, French SW: Dietary factors and alcoholic cirrhosis. *Alcoholism Clin Exp Res* 10:271-73, 1986.

54. Pryor WA, Lightsey JW, Prier DG: The production of free radicals in vivo from the action of xenobiotics: The initiation of autoxidation of polyunsaturated fatty acids by nitrogen dioxide and ozone, in Yagi K (ed): *Lipid Peroxides in Biology and Medicine.* Orlando, FL, Academic Press, 1982, p. 3.

55. Chang LW: Mercury, in Spencer PS, Schaumburg HH (eds): *Experimental and Clinical Neurotoxicology.* Williams and Wilkins, 1980, p. 522.

56. Levine SA, Kidd PM: *Antioxidant Adaptation: Its Role in Free Radical Pathology.* San Leandro, CA, Allergy Research Group, 1985, pp. 256-61.

57. Halliwell B. Gutteridge JMC: *Free Radicals in Biology and Medicine.* Oxford, Clarendon Press, 1985, p. 303.

58. Levine and Kidd, *Antioxidant Adaptation,* p. 278.

59. Ames B, Hollstein MC, Cathcart R: Lipid peroxidation and oxidative damage to DNA, in Yagi, *Lipid Peroxides,* p. 339.

60. Pryor et al, Production of free radicals, in Yagi, *Lipid Peroxides,* pp. 1-22.

61. Georgieff, KK: Free radical inhibitory effect of some anticancer compounds. *Science* 173:537-39, 1971.

62. Shamberger RJ, Baughman FF, Kalchert SL, et al: Carcinogen-induced chromosomal breakage decreased by antioxidants. *Proc Natl Acad Sci* 70:1461-63, 1973.

63. Black HS, Chan JT: Suppression of ultraviolet light-induced tumor formation by dietary antioxidants. *J Invest Dermatol* 65:412-14, 1975.

64. Cutler RG: Antioxidants and longevity, in Armstrong D, Sohal RS, Cutler RG, et al (eds): *Free Radicals in Molecular Biology, Aging and Disease.* New York, Raven Press, 1984, pp. 235-66.

65. Colditz GA, Branch LG, Lipnick RJ, et al: Increased green and yellow vegetable intake and lowered cancer deaths in an elderly population. *Am J Clin Nutr* 41:32-36, 1985.

66. Dayton S, Hashimoto S, Wollman J: Effect of high-oleic and high-linoleic safflower oils on mammary tumors induced in rats by 7, 12-dimethyl benz (alpha) anthracene. *J Nutr* 107:1353-60, 1977.

67. Broitman SA, Vitale JJ, Vavrousek-Jakuba E, et al: Poly-unsaturated fat, cholesterol and large bowel tumorigenesis. *Cancer* 40: 2455-63, 1977.

68. Kaneda J, Sakai H, Ishii S: Nutritive value or toxicity of highly unsaturated fatty acids, II. *J Biochem* 42:5, 561-73, 1955.

69. *Charaka Samhita,* vol. 2. Jamnagar, India, Shree Gulabkunverba Ayurvedic Society, 1949, sutrastana 27:293, p. 545.

70. Cohen LA, Thompson DO, Maeura Y, et al: Dietary fat and mammary cancer, 1. Promoting effects of different dietary fats on N-nitrosomethylurea-induced rat mammary tumorigenesis. *J Natl Canc Inst* 77:33-42, 1986.

71. Braden LM, Carroll KK: Dietary polyunsaturated fat in relation to mammary carcinogenesis in rats. *Lipids* 21:285-88, 1986.

72. Masi I, et al: Diets rich in saturated, monosaturated, and polyunsaturated fatty acids differently affect plasma lipids, platelet and arterial wall eicosanoids in rabbits. *Ann Nutr Metab* 30:66-72, 1986.

73. Reddy BS, Maruyama H: Effect of dietary fish oil on azoxymethane-induced colon carcinogenesis in male F344 rats. *Canc Res* 46:3367-70, 1986.

74. Harman D: Free radical theory of aging: Effect of the amount and degree of unsaturation of dietary fat on mortality rate. *J Gerontol* 26, no. 4:451-57, 1971.

75. Matsuo N: Studies on the toxicity of fish oil, II. *J Biochem* (Tokyo) 41:647-52, 1954.

76. Mead JF: Free radical mechanisms of lipid damage and consequences for cellular membranes, in Pryor WA (ed): *Free Radicals in Biology.* New York, Academic Press, 1976, pp. 51-68.

77. Ames BN: Dietary carcinogens and anticarcinogens, oxygen radicals and degenerative disease. *Science* 221:1256-63, 1983.

78. Rizek RL, Welsh SO, Marston RM, et al: Levels and sources of fat in the U.S. food supply and in diets of individuals, in Perkins and Visek, *Dietary Fats and Health,* pp. 13-43.

79. Torrielli MV, Dianzani MU: Free radicals in inflammatory disease, in Armstrong et al, *Free Radicals,* pp. 355-79.

80. Levine and Kidd, *Antioxidant Adaptation,* pp. 129-70.

81. Hirai S, Okamoto K, Morimatsu M: Lipid peroxide in the aging process, in Yagi, *Lipid Peroxides,* pp. 305-15.

82. Harman D: Free radicals and the origination, evolution and present status of the free radical theory of aging, in Armstrong et al, *Free Radicals,* pp. 1-12.

83. Pinckney ER: The potential toxicity of excessive polyunsaturates. *Am Heart J* 85, no. 6:723-26, 1973.

84. Yagi K: Assay for serum lipid peroxide level and its clinical significance, in Yagi, *Lipid Peroxides,* pp. 231-32.

85. Brisson, *Lipids in Human Nutrition,* p. 108.

86. Goto Y: Lipid peroxides as a cause of vascular diseases, in Yagi, *Lipid Peroxides,* pp. 295-303.

87. Harman D. Hendricks S, Eddy DE, Seibold J: Free radical theory of aging: Effect of dietary fat on central nervous system function. *J Am Geriatr Soc* 24, no. 7:301-7, 1976.

88. Nawar WW, Witchwoot A: Autoxidation of fats and oils at

elevated temperatures, in Simic MG, Karel M (eds): *Autoxidation in Food and Biological Systems.* New York, Plenum, 1980, pp. 207-21.

89. Billek G: Lipid stability and deterioration, in Perkins and Visek, *Dietary Fats and Health,* pp. 70-89.

90. Brisson, *Lipids in Human Nutrition,* pp. 31, 41.

91. Enig MG, Munn RJ, Keeney M: Dietary fat and cancer trends— a critique. *Federation Proceedings* 37:2215-20, 1978.

92. Clark AJ, van den Reek MM, Craig-Schmidt MC, Weete JD: Fat in the diets of adolescent girls with emphasis on isomeric fatty acids. *Am J Clin Nutr* 43:530-37, 1986.

93. Brewster L, Jacobson M: *The Changing American Diet.* Washington, DC, Center for Science in the Public Interest, 1983.

94. Kinsella JE, Bruckner G, Mai J, Shimp J: Metabolism of *trans* fatty acids with emphasis on the effects of *trans,* trans-octadecadienoate on lipid composition, essential fatty acid, and prostaglandins: An overview. *Am J Clin Nutr* 34:2307-18, 1981.

95. Watonabe M, Sugano M: Effects of dietary *cis-* and *trans-* monomene fats on 7, 12-dimethylbenz (a) anthracene-induced rat mammary tumors. *Nutr Reps Internatl* 33, no. 1:163-69, 1986.

96. Brisson, *Lipids in Human Nutrition,* pp. 41-71.

97. Kritchevsky D: Influence of *trans* unsaturated fat on experimental atherosclerosis, in Perkins and Visek, *Dietary Fats and Health,* pp. 404-6.

98. Wellcome Foundation: Interferon production. *Chem Abstracts* 90:157072f, 1979.

99. Wara E, Pockl E, Mullner E, Wintersberger E: Effect of sodium butyrate on induction of cellular and viral DNA syntheses in polyoma virus-infected mouse kidney cells. *J Virol* 38, no. 3:973-81, 1981.

100. Taki T, Hirabayashi Y, Kondo R: Effect of butyrate on glycolipid metabolism of two cell types of rat ascites hepatomas with different ganglioside biosynthesis. *J Biochem* 96:1395-1402, 1979.

101. Cousens LS, Gallwitz D, Alberts BM: Different accessibilities in chromatin to histone acetylase. *J Bio Chem* 254, no. 5:1716-23, 1979.

102. Borenfreund E, Schmid E, Bendich A, et al: Constitutive aggregates of intermediate-sized filaments of the vimentin and cytokeratin type in cultured hepatoma cells and their dispersal by butyrate. *Exp Cell Res* 127:215-35, 1980.

103. Bradford RW, Allen HW, Culbert ML: *Butyric Acid Therapy as a New Adjunctive in the Treatment of Degenerative Diseases.* Chula Vista, CA, Bradford Research Institute, 1983.

104. Tallman JF, Smith CC, Henneberry RC: Induction of functional beta-adrenergic receptors in HeLa cells. *Proc Natl Sci USA* 74, no. 3:873-77, 1977.

105. Mitkov D, Toreva D: A study on the comatose action of short chain fatty acids. *Folia Medica* (Plovdiv) 21:20-24, 1979.

106. Fisk AA: Senile dementia, Alzheimer-type (SDAT): A review of present knowledge. *Wisc Med J* 78:29-33, 1979.

107. Yajima T, Kojima K. Tohyama K, Mutai M: Effect of short-chain fatty acids on electrical activity of the small intestinal mucosa of rat. *Life Sciences* 28:983-89, 1981.

108. Terry RD, Davies P: Dementia of the Alzheimer type. *Ann Rev Neuroscience* 3:77-95, 1980.

109. Simmons JL, Fishman PH, Freese E, Brady RO: Morphological alterations and ganglioside sialyltransferase activity induced by small fatty acids in HeLa cells. *J Cell Biol* 66:414-24, 1975.

110. Robert W. Bradford, Robert W. Bradford Research Institute, Chula Vista, CA, telephone conversation with author, 26 Jan 1987.

111. Price WA: *Nutrition and Physical Degeneration.* Santa Monica, CA, Price-Pottenger Nutrition Foundation, 1975, p. 438.

112. Ballentine RM: *Diet and Nutrition.* Honesdale, PA, Himalayan Institute, 1978, pp. 465-66.

113. Ames BN: Dietary carcinogens and anticarcinogens. *Science* 221:1256-62, 1983.

114. Rechcigl M: *Handbook of Naturally Occurring Food Toxicants.* Boca Raton, FL, CRC Press, 1983.

115. Mettlin C: Epidemiologic findings relating diet to cancer of the esophagus, in Reddy and Cohen, *Diet, Nutrition, and Cancer,* vol. 2, p. 84.

116. Anderson K, Kies C: Nitrate and nitrite excretion in weanling rats as affected by dietary fiber, in Hemphill DD (ed): *Trace Substances in Environmental Health XVII.* Columbia, MO, University of Missouri, 1983.

117. Smith LL: The autoxidation of cholesterol, in Simic MG, Karel M: *Autoxidation in Food and Biological Systems.* New York, Plenum Press, 1980, pp. 119-32.

118. Peng SK, Taylor CB: Atherogenic effect of oxidized cholesterol, in Perkins EG, Visek WJ (eds): *Dietary Fats and Health.* Champaign, IL, American Oil Chemists' Society, 1983, pp. 919-33.

119. Jacobson MS, Price MG, Shamoo AE, Heald FP: Atherogenesis in the white Carneau pigeons: Effects of low-level cholestane-triol feeding. *Atherosclerosis* 57:209-17, 1985.

120. Sheppard AJ, Shen CJ: Activities of FDA's division of nutrition regarding cholesterol oxides, in Simic and Karel, *Autoxidation in Food and Biological Systems,* pp. 133-40.

121. Jacobson MS: Cholesterol oxides in Indian ghee: Possible cause of unexplained high risk of atherosclerosis in Indian immigrant populations. *Lancet* 19 Sep 1987, 656-58.

122. Malhotra S: Epidemiology of ischemic heart disease in India with special reference to causation. *Brit Heart J* 29:895-905, 1967.

Commentarial Notes

nt. 1 In the middle range, defined by the ellipse, the correlation is actually reversed: the ellipse tilts in the opposite direction from the line.

In that middle range, most populations with higher cholesterol intakes have *less* heart disease. This is probably because in this moderate range cholesterol itself does not play a major role. Instead, other factors that happen to be more extreme come to be of overriding importance in determining the incidence of heart disease. For example, the unusually low levels of soil selenium in Finland have been thought to contribute to heart disease. Perhaps in France and Switzerland there are factors related to diet, lifestyle, or heredity that are protective. As we shall see later in this chapter, butter in the diet, which increases cholesterol intake, may actually play some protective role vis-à-vis heart disease.

nt. 2 A mixture of *Lactobacillus bulgaricas* and *Lactobacillus acidophilus* is probably preferable.

nt. 3 While the issue of the etiology of immune disorders is presently under intensive investigation and there are many diverging views, it is certainly possible to make a good case for the importance of psychological factors in determining the severity and direction of hyperimmune phenomena such as allergies.[28]

nt. 4 The studies cited that show a correlation between multiple sclerosis and milk consumption are based on studies of populations wherein milk is not boiled before use. Figures for the countries of southern Asia, where boiling is the custom, are not available.

nt. 5 The Helsinki study[41] showed a reduction in heart disease in men, but none for women. The Oslo study[43] showed a reduction in deaths from heart disease at 5 years, but by 11 years the difference had disappeared.

nt. 6 Pooling the data from the four studies eliminated any statistically significant differences in cancer incidence and mortality.[46] That was accomplished, however, by adding in the data from those studies wherein heart disease was not reduced by the dietary intervention. It remains true that in the one study in which there was a good response in terms of the reduction of heart disease there *was* a significant concomitant rise in cancer rates.

nt. 7 Traditionally sesame oil, which is only partially unsaturated, was considered the safest[69] (and safflower oil, the most highly polyunsaturated, the least desirable). Olive oil, which is another oil that is not unsaturated to a high degree, has recently been reported to be associated with a lowered incidence of some tumors[70] (rather than a higher incidence, as is the case with other vegetable oils). Recent studies suggest that oils high in linolenic acid do not have the same carcinogenic potential as those high in linoleic acid.[71] Olive oil is also increasingly found to have a favorable effect on blood lipids.[72]

Fish oils, though they are also highly unsaturated, have not behaved like vegetable oils in experiments done on cancer promotion in animals,[73] nor have they decreased longevity, as have vegetable oils.[74]

Yet studies in the past have reported some toxic effects from fish oils that are similar to those of polyunsaturated oils from vegetable sources.[75] And some authors are still expressing concern about the effects of such oils.[76,77]

nt. 8 Such a diagrammatic representation of a complex biological interplay will inevitably involve some oversimplification. For example there is evidence that some of the well-known antioxidants that help prevent free radical propogation, such as vitamin C, are not associated with increased longevity (though most are).[64]

nt. 9 It's been estimated that trans-fatty acids constitute 7% to 10% of the averages person's intake,[91] though one recent survey[92] showed only 6.5% in the current American diet. Although estimates vary, because of the increase in consumption of margarines and vegetable shortenings it seems likely that intake has increased by a factor of three to five in the last 70 years.[93]

nt. 10 This point is highly controversial. Enig's conclusions have been widely criticized. One recent study done with experimental animals showed no difference between cis- and trans-fatty acids in their effects on tumor incidence.[95]

nt. 11 The whole critique of trans-fatty acids is currently the subject of heated debate. A helpful review of the subject is found in Brisson.[96]

nt. 12 This information has been synthesized by Dr. Robert Bradford,[110] who has summarized it in a recent report.[103] The basic documentation[104-9] is given here, since the concept will be unfamiliar to most readers and therefore its thesis may seem unwarranted.

nt. 13 As an unsaturated lipid, cholesterol is susceptible to free radical oxidation in the presence of air.[117] The resulting oxides of cholesterol have been found to be toxic to the cells lining the arteries of rabbits[118] and birds[119] and thus suspected of being one of the initiating factors in human atherosclerosis (as well as being carcinogenic).[120] On a recent analysis of ghee samples an average of 12% of the cholesterol was present as oxides, an amount thought to be sufficient to damage arterial linings, and the author of the report suggests that the use of ghee might account for the higher risk of heart disease observed in Indian immigrants.[121] However, epidemiologic studies done in India 20 years ago showed a sevenfold higher incidence of heart disease in South Indians who used little or no ghee, compared with Punjabis who used large amounts.[122] Moreover, the truth is, most Indians don't use clarified butter these days anyway. They use "vegetable ghee," which is hydrogenated vegetable oil. While these points throw considerable doubt on the hypothesis that ghee causes heart attacks, one must still be concerned about the discovery of cholesterol oxides in it. In this connection, several additional points might be considered:

1. Ghee may be prepared (especially that available commercially) from rancid butter, the cholesterol of which may already have undergone oxidation.
2. The method of preparation of the ghee may have been faulty. For example, copper pots are apparently used at times,[121] which is not advisable (nor is it condoned in the Ayurvedic tradition) because copper might catalyze cholesterol oxidation.
3. If cholesterol oxides do turn out to be present in properly prepared ghee, precisely which ones are produced will require careful scrutiny. It is thought that the most toxic of these compounds are cholestane triol and 25 hydroxycholesterol.[118] In the assay mentioned above,[121] the first of these was found only in trace amounts, while the second was not measured separately from a third compound.

Though at this point in time the angiotoxicity of vegetable oils seems more firmly established than that of carefully made ghee, it seems increasingly obvious that it is desirable to keep the use of fats and oils of all sorts in cooking at levels much lower than is presently common.

Moreover, while the role of cholesterol oxides in the causation of atherosclerosis is being more fully explored, it is prudent to avoid foods known to contain large amounts of the more toxic of these compounds, such as powdered custard and pancake mixes, cheeses stored at room temperature, foods fried in repeatedly used animal fats such as lard, and (of a lower order of toxicity, but perhaps of greater concern) powdered infant milk formulas.[118] There are also sterols in plant foods that may be likewise sensitive to oxidation. Perhaps this line of research will result in a greater appreciation of the freshness of food as a critical factor in diet.

nt. 14 Before use, containers should be washed well to remove grease that adheres and protects microbes, and then exposed to hot water, preferably scalding. Those containers made of plastic almost seem designed to spread the growth of microorganisms, since plastic develops tiny nicks and scratches where bacteria can thrive. The scratches and crevices in the plastic also make thorough cleaning difficult, and it can't be put in boiling water. But, if it is well scrubbed with detergent to remove all grease, plastic can be soaked in a solution of laundry bleach and water, which will disinfect it. But there remains the risk of food picking up chemicls from plastic containers, which give it an off-taste and may adversely affect the food or the person who eats it. For such reasons plastic containers are less than ideal for storing cooked food. Glass is excellent, but glass is not very practical because it's easily broken. Probably the best choice currently is the stainless steel container with a plastic snap cap. (The plastic need not come in contact with the food.) Plastic wrap can also be used as a cover, but the containers should be well sealed, since even when a refrigerator is clean, the food will deteriorate from exposure to air. Although it is not necessary to vacuum-pack leftovers to store them for a couple of days, oxidation can be reduced by putting the food in containers that can be closed tightly and that are the correct size so that they contain little air.

nt. 15 A recent report suggests that spinach, because of its fiber content, also has the capacity to pick up toxic nitrites and carry them out of the body.[116] For this reason a small amount of darkened leaf is probably harmless, but if spoilage proceeds, it probably reaches a point where the amount of nitrites resulting exceeds the binding capacity of the vegetable, and the spinach becomes a liability.

The Vegetarian Diet in Perspective: An Overview

Citational Notes

1. Freeland-Graves JH, Bodzy PW, Eppright MA: Zinc status of vegetarians. *J Am Dietetic Assn* 77:655-61, 1980.

2. Abdulla M, Aly KO, Andersson I, et al: Nutrient intake and health status of lactovegetarins. *Am J Clin Nutr* 40:325-38, 1984.

3. U.S. Department of Agriculture: *Nutrient Intakes: Individuals in 48 States, Year 1977-78.* Nationwide Food Consumption Survey, 1977-78, Report no. 1-2, 1984.

4. Stamler J: Population Studies, in Levy RI, et al (eds): *Nutrition, Lipids, and Coronary Heart Disease: A Global View.* New York, Raven Press, 1979, p. 57.

INDEX

Antioxidants: and free radical
inactivation, 216-18; and longevity,
218-19, 287nt.8; spices as, 233
Arthritis: and calcium metabolism,
126; and free radical damage, 217
Arachidonic acid: in cell membranes,
quantity as compared with
eicosapentaenoic acid (EPA), and
blood clotting, 151-52; as an
essential fatty acid, 149
Aspergillus flavus, growth on peanuts,
106
Asthma and milk allergy, 206
Atherosclerosis, 49-53. *See also* Heart
disease
—and calcium metabolism, 126
—and cardiovascular disease, 49-53
—causal factors proposed: free radical
damage, 219; cholesterol oxides in
ghee, 287-88nt.13; difficulty of
studying when prevalent in
population, 190-91; irritation of
arterial linings by vegetable oils as
initiating factor, 219-20; molecular
clutter in tissues, 195-96; zinc
deficiency, 136
—and consumption of: butterfat, 211;
fats and oils, 50; fish, 143; fish oil,
145-47
—prevention and/or treatment:
through diet, 51-52, 192-93; use of
legumes in, 97; role of pectin in,
199-200
—tissue changes in, 49
Athletic performance and meat
consumption, 19-20
Ayurvedic teachings relative to ghee,
225

Bacterial contamination of meat,
poultry, fish, milk. *See* Meat,
Poultry, Fish, Milk, bacterial
contamination of
Bacterial digestion of cellulose in
colon, 200
Bacterial flora of the gut: as a source

of vitamin B_{12}, 170-73; as consumer
of vitamin B_{12}, 171-72
Bacterial growth in the intestinal tract,
effects of yogurt consumption on,
205
Balanced diet, vegetarian, design of,
227-31. *See also* Nutritional
requirements
Bean balls recipe, 77
Beans. *See* Legumes
Beans and rice: and the prevention of
atherosclerotic heart disease, 52-53,
97; ratios for optimal protein
quality, 95-96
Behavioral problems from milk
consumption by lactose-intolerant
children, 204
Beta carotene as a free radical
inactivator, 216-18
Bible and vegetarianism, 6
Bile acids and cancer, 47
Bile salts: definition, 192; as route of
excretion for cholesterol, 192-93
Birth defects and maternal manganese
deficiency, 133
Bleeding problems: among Eskimos
consuming diets high in fish, 148-
49; from excess eicosapentaenoic
acid (EPA) capsules, 148, 277nt.2
Bloating from vegetarian diet, 201
Blood pressure. *See* High blood
pressure
Boiling milk, reasons for and
importance of, 207-9
Bone deposition promoters, 128
Bone loss: in Eskimos, 122; as the
price of calcium balance in meat-
eaters, 271nt.16; in vegetarians as
compared with meat-eaters, 122-25.
See also Osteoporosis
Bone mass, peak and susceptibility to
osteoporosis, 114-15
Bone mineralization and vitamin D,
116-17
Bran: basic components of, 199; as
dietary supplement: pros and cons,